A GOOD HEALTH GUIDE

Clean Your Liver

Maxwell Stein

Clean Your Liver

Maxwell Stein

This edition published MMI by The Bristol Group Ltd,
158 Moulsham Street,
Chelmsford,
Essex CM2 0LD

Typeset by SJ Design and Publishing, Bromley, Kent

ISBN 1-903904-04-8

Contents

Introduction

Clean Your Liver is loosely based on the Chinese philosophy of Yin and Yang. There are two characteristics which complement and balance each other. Yin or 'shade' represents the feminine or cooler force which is the flexible yielding side of nature. Yang or 'sunlight' is the hotter, stronger and more positive force. Everyone has these two elements in combination as do most foods which can also be categorised as Yin or Yang. This programme is aimed at balancing the two in the right way for each individual. It is a balance of foods adapted to suit the different needs and tastes of each individual.

What I have found has astounded me. I can't believe it has taken me this long. The liver is the supreme organ of metabolism. It has to be the missing key to unlock the problems of obesity. People who are more calm, relaxed, peaceful, creative and social are said to contain a higher proportion of Yin. Their preference is to eat salads and fruits. Those who are more Yang are active and alert, are energetic and precise. They prefer hotter, spicier foods.

The aim therefore, is to balance the Yin and Yang by first cleansing the body of impurities and then adjust the Yin and Yang to complement the individual person.

The Complete Liver Cleansing Programme in Chapter 3 has been developed for you to study and carry out in a correct and controlled manner. It is essential, therefore, that all who participate should appreciate its importance and have a firm belief in it.

It is evident, of course, that the student who has faith in The Complete Liver Cleansing Programme will devote his/her mind to its study, and practice its discipline with enthusiasm, perseverance and pleasure. The student should choose an hour or so, preferably when not too tired, to sit comfortably and digest the information from within these pages and to enjoy the relaxation of doing so.

It is of the greatest import to the success of *Clean Your Liver* that the student has confidence in the programme.

The liver is a complex organ. Its structure embraces all the basics of bio-engineering, and its chemical fluids and secretions are finely balanced. It is not an organ to be abused. The liver is the 'Commander-in-Chief' taking charge of all health functions. It is the liver which stores the blood and adjusts its supply to meet the body's needs. Its vitally connected with the purification of your entire system, the correct processing of protein, liquids and foods. Plus importantly it controls your metabolism.

Before starting the programme, the student should know broadly how the body is going to respond to the changes in attitude and diet; the student must therefore know something about the physiology of the liver. By having a knowledge of how the liver works the student is able to make informed decisions in understanding the problems the liver is encountering. By a familiarity with the nutritional benefits of food, he/she will be primed to investigate with advantage, the nutritional properties and uses of foodstuffs from any part of the world, and to use and apply them as remedial means for his/her own benefit.

It is important to note that only reasonably fit and healthy people should take part in The Complete Liver Cleansing Programme. Those who should definitely not take part are people with diabetes, epilepsy, anaemia or wasting diseases such as cancer, leukaemia or TB. People who become light-headed or develop headaches when they miss a meal could have a blood sugar problem, so they should not take part, neither should people who tire easily. These groups should consult their practitioner for diagnosis and advice.

WARNING

The contents of this book have been carefully checked for accuracy. The reader is advised that the information contained herein may not be representative of health professionals and physicians and must not be looked upon as a substitute for professional advice from a qualified practitioner.

As a general precaution, women should seek professional advice before taking any of the treatments mentioned during pregnancy.

Neither the author or the publishers can accept legal responsibility for any problems that may arise out of experimentation with any of the methods, recommendations or suggestions described within this book.

Chapter 1

The Physiology of Your Liver

Inside your body, located behind the lower ribs on the right side of your abdominal cavity, lies the liver. It is attached to the *diaphragm* by *ligaments* which hold it in place. When you breath deeply, the liver rolls forward and downwards, and can be felt through the *abdominal wall.* The liver is completely covered by the *peritoneum* except at a point where it is held along the line of attachment to the *ligaments*.

It is the largest and one of the most complex organs in your body. Its healthy function fulfills an important role in maintaining and controlling the processes necessary to the existence of human life.

The liver is divided into four parts, called *lobes,* with the right *lobe* much larger than the others. Each *lobe* contains as many as 100,000 smaller *lobes,* known as *lobules.* These *lobules* are six-sided cells arranged in layers one cell thick, and are closely arranged around *lymph vessels*, *blood vessels*, *bile ducts,* and *nerves*. Certain *reticuloendothelial cells (Kupffer cells)* line these *lobules* and play a role in immunity.

It is normal for three sides of each cell to be in contact with a *blood vessel,* and the other three adjacent to a *bile duct.* The *lobules* are grouped in clusters so that the *bile* manufactured by each *lobule* passes down a common duct, which links to larger ducts that connects to the common *hepatic duct.* This duct joins with the *cystic duct* of the *gall bladder* and goes into the *duodenum* along with the *pancreatic duct* of *Wirsung.* Once in the *intestines*, *bile salts* help to emulsify fats and enhance the *metabolism* of *fats* and *proteins* by *enzymes.*

The liver is a highly vascular organ. It is served by two separate blood supplies. The *hepatic artery* supplies 25% of its blood. The other 75% comes from the *portal vein,* which transports digested nutrients and hormones from the *intestines,* hormones from the *pancreas*, and old *red blood cells* and *bilirubin,* a component of *bile*, from the *spleen.* Blood leaves the liver via the *hepatic veins* and thence to the *inferior vena cava* and the *heart.* About half a litre of blood remains in the liver at all times.

The weight of an adult males liver is between 1.5 to 1.8 kg in weight and is slightly less than this in women. It is asymmetric in shape and is a dark reddish-brown colour. Its texture is soft, but firm.

Researchers have identified more that 500 different functions of the liver. Several of the major functions are for processing compounds used by the body which include *hæmoglobin*, *glucose*, *vitamins, proteins* and *fats.*

To fulfill the many functions it is called upon by the body to do, it is necessary for the liver to be in peak condition at all times.

FUNCTIONS OF YOUR LIVER

This vital organ performs many complex functions, but its primary functions are:

- □ To produce and export important chemical substances used by the rest of the body.
- □ To convert the food we eat into stored energy and to control the release of that energy when it is required. The liver also converts food into essential chemicals for growth and to maintain a good healthy life.
- □ To process drugs and medications taken in from the *digestive tract* and convert them into substances that are easier for the body to assimilate. Thus enabling the body to use them more competently and to dispose of the waste products from them.
- □ To act as a filter to detoxify and eliminate from the body, substances that would otherwise be poisonous.
- □ To manufacture important body chemicals, one of which is the production of *bile*, which is supplied to the *gall bladder* and is necessary for the digestion of foods.
- □ To decide which substances are to be stored and transformed into chemicals suitable for the body to assimilate.

HOW YOUR LIVER SUPPORTS YOUR BODILY FUNCTIONS:

- □ By producing energy fast, when it is needed.
- □ By manufacturing proteins necessary for the body to grow. Proteins are found everywhere in nature, and no life form can survive without them. *Proteins* are fabricated by simple organic compounds, the *amino acids*, which contain *nitrogen* and from time to time *sulphur*. Humans build the *proteins* that they need for

growth and repair of tissues by breaking down the proteins acquired in food, into their fundamental parts, the *amino acids*, and then building up the components into *proteins* of the type required. Animal sources provide *protein-rich* foods which contain complete proteins, these supply all *the amino acids* in the proper proportions necessary in the human diet. To obtain proteins from plant life we must obtain a mixture of plants to get the proper complement of *amino acids*, an all important matter of concern to vegetarians.

□ By controlling the storage and movement of fat within the body. Fats that are broadly disbursed in nature, are a concentrated food source of energy. Fats are *glyceryl esters* of fatty acids and produce *glycerol* and many other different fatty acids when broken down by *hydrolysis*.

□ By storing *vitamins*, *sugars* and *minerals* and releasing them to the body when called upon. Surplus nutrients not immediately used to meet energy requirements are stored in a carbohydrate reserve called *glycogen* and in a fat reserve called *triglyceride*, stored in *adipose tissue*.

□ By controlling the clotting of blood. Many body proteins are manufactured by the liver such as *albumin*, and blood clotting factors such as *prothrombin* and *fibronogen* that cause the blood to clot when needed.

□ By controlling the manufacture and excretion of cholesterol. It is derived from foods that are saturated with fatty acids, it is also manufactured biosynthetically from *acetate*, which is primarily in the liver.

□ *Cholesterol* is the forerunner of the bile acids in the liver.

There are 24 *steroid carboxylic* acids that aid in the digestion of foods, especially *lipids*, and, when combined with the *amino acids glycine* or *taurine*, form the *bile salts*. The synthesis of *cholesterol* in the liver is under feedback control, therefore the total amount of *cholesterol* from these two sources remains constant. Synthesis increases when the dietary intake is low, and low when the dietary intake is high.

- □ The *blood* transports dietary *cholesterol* from the *intestines* to the liver via large *lipoprotein* molecules known as *chylomicrons.* The liver then secretes *Very Low Density Lipoprotein* containing *cholesterol* and *cholesterol ester* into the *blood.*
- □ Low Density Lipoproteins are the result of *very Low Density Lipoproteins* being partially converted in *adipose tissue. Low Density Lipoproteins* are the primary carrier *proteins* for *cholesterol,* supplying both *free* and *esterified cholesterol* to the divers body tissues. *High Density Lipoproteins* are involved in the conveyance of *cholesterol* to the liver where it is broken down and excreted, it also removes some of the *Low Density Lipoproteins* from the walls of the *arteries.*

By synthesising and disposing of unwanted poisonous substances.

- □ By metabolising alcohol. Most of the alcohol that is drunk is metabolised by the liver. Small amounts are secreted as urine after being processed by the *kidneys,* and a small amount is processed through the *lungs* and exhaled in the breath.

- By monitoring the blood as it circulates through the liver, and correcting the level of the many chemicals, proteins and drugs called upon by the body.
- By cleansing the blood of all waste products before it is returned reinvigorated to the body.
- By maintaining and correcting hormonal equilibrium. Human *hormones* are often constrained to *blood proteins*, which protect the *hormones* from premature degradation. In the case of *steroid hormones*, they become more soluble in a fluid medium. The duration that a single *hormone* molecule can circulate in the *blood* is short, and can range from minutes to hours. The concentration of a circulating *hormone* is influenced by the *metabolism*, the uptake, and the disregard of the circulating *hormone* by target tissues, the liver, and *excretory organs*.
- By serving as the main organ of *blood* development in the *womb* before birth.
- By the manufacture of chemicals to help the body to resist infection by producing immune factors and by removing *bacteria* from the *blood stream.*
- By storing iron throughout life. Minerals, such as iron are essential to life and health. They are an essential part of all cells and body fluids and enter into many physiological and anatomical functions.
- By regenerating its own tissues to replace those that have been damaged. If a disease progresses beyond the tissue's capacity to regenerate new cells, the body's entire metabolism is severely affected.

Almost everything we eat and drink must pass through our liver. It is essential therefore to give careful thought and attention to our diet. Proper nutrition is vital to the well-being and maintenance of a good healthy liver and consequently to the rest of our body.

Chapter 2

Taking Control of Your Metabolism

Metabolism can be described as 'the sum of all the chemical change reactions in the living cell that are used for the production of useful work and the synthesis of cell constituents'. In short, it is the process of growth and maintenance of the body, and is brought about by the ceaseless chemical and physical changes and modifications that take place. Once the nutrients have entered the bloodstream and lymphatic vessels, absorption is complete and metabolism begins. Nutrients thus supply the molecules from which energy, as calories, may be derived for cellular synthesis, cell and organ growth, and tissue replacement. In Chinese medicine the liver is described as the 'Zang' organ and is responsible for the smooth flow of energy (Qi) and blood throughout the body.

The minimal requirements of energy required by the human body is expressed in terms of calories, which are units of heat. For every gram of pure protein that is ingested, it will yield 4 calories, one gram of pure fat will yield nine calories, and one gram of pure carbohydrate will yield four calories.

THE CORRECT APPROACH TO CALORIES

The amount of energy used each day depends on the type

of activity carried out, and upon the individuals metabolism. A slightly built person doing a comparatively sedate activity throughout the day will use as little as 2000 calories a day, whilst an 80kg person doing hard physical labour throughout the day will burn twice as much. However, the equation is not that simple, people with a fast metabolic rate usually burn up more calories than those who are calm.

At a reasonable level of activity, the average person's calorie requirement is considered to be around 2000 to 3000 calories per day. Never allow your calorie intake to go below 1000 calories per day, unless of course you are dieting under medical supervision.

PROTEINS AND THEIR ORIGINS

Proteins form the building blocks of the basic structure of tendons, nails, hair, muscles, bones and other tissues. We need about 40g to 50g of proteins per day to repair and maintain damaged tissues and generate new ones to take their place. A protein molecule contains *nitrogen, oxygen, carbon* and *hydrogen* atoms, and not infrequently *phosphorus* and *sulpher* atoms.

The liver needs a good supply of protein for greatest proficiency. Milk protein is the finest form of protein suitable for the liver, we can benefit from proteins taken in the form of curds, yoghurt, sour milk or cottage cheese. Almonds contain high quality protein. Almost 25% of its bulk is made up of protein. Soya beans are also an excellent source of protein. Wheat germ is greatly valued as a protein grain.

The *amino acids* in protein have to be in certain combinations before the body can assimilate them. Various animal foods such as eggs, cheese, meat and milk all have the right mixture but also have a lot of fat, it is better therefore to use plant protein. Pulses, beans peas, lentils, wheat and oats all include protein but require to be combined to furnish the right mixture of *amino acids.*

IMPROVING YOUR DIGESTION

Food should be a delight to the senses. Eating, whether it is a home cooked meal or dining at our favourite restaurant or having a snack between meals; it should always be a satisfying experience. All the food that we eat must eventually be processed by the liver into suitable chemicals and compounds. It is therefore the responsibility of the individual to regulate the amount of essential and non essential foods that are ingested. Failure to recognise and act upon these facts will undoubtedly cause the breakdown of some of the body's normal functions. This will result in the misery of ill-health.

Fortunately, changing our diet for the benefit of good health, or to become slim and body beautiful, is not a chore. To maintain our body in tip-top condition it is only necessary to eat the right food in the right amounts to keep the body supplied with the correct amount of nutrition. This does not mean that we have to eat dull uninspiring food. With all the varied and delicious foods available to us, thanks to modern technology, and the information provided on the properties within these foods, we now have a multiplicity of choice in selecting good healthy foods essential to a good healthy liver, and consequently a healthy body.

In the following chapters *Clean Your Liver* will show you which of these healthy foods to eat, when to eat them and how to cook them. Remember, it is your diet in its entirety that is important; not just for today, but for the rest of your life!

CHOOSING WHICH FOODS TO EAT

It is important that we eat a wide variety of foods to ensure an adequate supply of vitamins and minerals in our diet. This is because while some nutrients tend to be found in abundant quantities in certain groups of food, other nutrients are found in lesser quantities in a much larger range of food. If we make a wise choice from a large variety of foods we are less likely to miss out on any one particular nutrient. However, it is important to know something about the contents of the food that we eat. Once we know what we are consuming then a decision can be made whether or not to keep them in our diet.

RID YOUR BODY OF FAT

Much has been said and written about the different types of fat contained in our food. Current opinion is this. Change your eating habits by consuming less than 30% of your daily calories in the form of fats.

There are many different types of fat which go to make up the fat in foods; these are called *fatty acids*. Depending on their chemical structure they can be described as either saturated fat or unsaturated fat.

Saturated Fats

Saturated fats originate mostly from animal products and are found in meats, dairy produce and some margarines. They are usually hard at room temperature.

Unsaturated Fats

Unsaturated fats are mostly liquid or oils and are found mostly in vegetables or are extracted as oils from various plants.

Monounsaturated Fats

This is a fat or oil obtained from one single source of vegetable or plant.

Polyunsaturated Fats

This is the from the same sources as monounsaturated fats but is a blend of different fats and oils from vegetables and plants.

DAIRY PRODUCTS

To reach a healthy low calorie diet leave the full cream milk on the supermarket shelf and use skimmed or semi-skimmed milk. Instead of choosing cream or soured cream buy low fat natural yoghurt or fromage frais. If sweetening is necessary add a little honey. Needless to say, if we change the product to improve our nutrition then the taste of the substitute will be different; this is a fact of life. It is however, a very small sacrifice to make when considering the enormous benefits a good diet can bring to our mental and physical well-being.

It is not good to drink with your meals. Excessive intake of liquid dilutes the gastric juices and therefore slows down the digestive process. Much better to drink a glass of water half an hour before your meal and then a glass of fruit or vegetable juice half an hour after you have eaten.

For a healthier liver and consequently a healthier body, it is important to decrease the amount of fat in our food and to change to the less saturated fat. The chart below shows a range of popular dairy products that are consumed in our everyday diet and are either high or low in saturated fat. If we are to enjoy the food we eat we should know what we are eating. Get to know what is good for you and your body will reward you amply. The easy way to find dietary information about the foods we buy is to read the information on the food wrapping. After all, we have fought to make the manufacturers declare these facts, so its a good idea to make use of the information provided.

Dairy Products	**g/100g**	**Dairy Products**	**g/100g**
Cheddar cheese	34g	Low fat natural yoghurt	2g
Stilton cheese	35g	Greek yoghurt	21g
Full fat soft cheese	42g	Low fat single cream	9g
Cream cheese	47g	Low fat double cream	24g
Low fat cottage cheese	1.8g	Half cream	12g
Cottage cheese	4g	Sour cream	18g
Curd cheese	12g	Single cream	18g
Low fat cheese	15g	Whipping cream	35g
Camembert cheese	23g	Double cream	48g
Skinned milk	0.1g	Quark	1g

Dairy Products	g/100g	Dairy Products	g/100g
Semi-skinned milk	1.6g	Very low fat spreads	28g
Whole milk	3.9g	Low fat spreads	40g
Evaporated milk	9g	Reduced low fat spread	60g
Sweetened condensed milk	9g	Margarine (including Polyunsaturated margarine)	80g
Fromage frais	0.2g		
Buttermilk	0.1g	Butter	82g

Figures represent grams of fat in every 100g of the product

MEAT

Most cuts of meat contain a lot of saturated fat. Cut the fat off meat and remove the skin from poultry. When sealing meat for a casserole use a dry non-stick pan instead of browning in hot fat. If making casseroles with pre-cooked meat or with meat stock, allow the casserole to cool and remove the fat that has risen to the surface. When cooking stews or soups leave out the traditional thickening agents which are full of fats. Use instead puréed vegetables, the improvement in taste and nutrition is stunning. Joints cooked in the oven should be place on a trivet so that the fat can be discarded.

Product	g/100g	Product	g/100g
Bacon (fried)	40.6	Lamb (roast)	17.9
Bacon (grilled)	33.8	Pork (roast)	19.8
Bacon, Streaky (Fried)	44.8	Turkey (roast)	4.1
Bacon, Streaky (grilled)	36.0	Venison (roast)	6.4
Rump Steak (fried)	14.6	Ham (roast)	22.1
Rump Steak (grilled)	12.1	Goose (roast)	22.4

Chicken, (boiled)	9.9	Beef (minced)	15.2
Frankfurters	25.0	Sausages (pork)	24.6

Figures represent grams of fat in every 100g of the product.

ROASTING AND GRILLING

When roasting use polyunsaturated oil instead of hard fats, quite often less is required. Instead of frying use a grill pan or better still use a grill.

FRYING

Potato chips seem to be a world-wide favourite. Here is one product that can still be enjoyed on occasions without having to change the way in which it is cooked. Always use an oil that is high in polyunsaturates and cook them at a high temperature, they will cook more quickly and will not soak up the oil. Avoid making thin and crinkle-cut chips. The smaller the surface area the less fat taken up. When removing from the oil, allow the excess oil to drip back into the pan. Drain the chips on a bed of kitchen paper, to absorb any remaining oil.

CONTROL YOUR INTAKE OF SUGAR

There are two types of sugar, *fructose* and *monosaccharides*, which includes *glucose*, or *dextrose* as it is sometimes called. *Fructose* is the pure sugar gained from fruits, and can be obtained from health food shops. *Monosaccharides* is the sugar that usually ends up in your sugar bowl. This is an extract from sugar beets or sugar cane. It is a commercial white sugar, either in powder or granulated form. This sugar has gone through the processes of blending and refining for marketing in various forms.

You could manage to get along with no intake of sugar at all. It provides plenty of calories but no other nutrients. There is also three problems with eating sugar. First it tempts you to eat more than is necessary. That is why so much sugar is put into commercial foods and in chocolate and sweets and fizzy drinks. Secondly it is the main cause of tooth decay and gum disorders. Third and foremost, any excess refined sugar that is ingested will be converted into fats such as *cholesterol* and *triglycerides*, which will build up inside the cells and will eventually cause the functional deterioration of our *arteries* and also our organs such as the *heart,* liver and *kidneys.*

Try to avoid eating large amounts of sugar. Reduce the amount of sugar in your tea or coffee. To sweeten home cooked cakes use dried fruits such as dates, raisins, currants or sultanas; they also make ideal sweeteners for puddings. Honey is also a good substitute for sugar. It is more beneficial than refined sugar as it contains many trace elements used by our bodies and it takes the digestive system longer to absorb.

CONTROL YOUR INTAKE OF WATER

Water comprises about 66% of the body's weight. Without realising we rarely drink sufficient water to satisfy the needs of our body. Life as we know it cannot exist without water. If we sweat, we lose water out of the pores of our skin, this triggers the sensation of thirst; this is our body telling us that we need more water to maintain our bodily functions.

On close examination we find that there are numerous minerals in water that our body can render to good use. On the other hand, water supplied through pipes between the reservoir and the tap can contain contaminants from the chemicals used to 'purify' the water. There are however, no calories in water. Under normal circumstances our bodily need for fresh water is about 2 litres per day. Fresh water helps to cleanse the liver and kidneys. If you are slimming it will also help with weight loss. In addition to drinking water, eat plenty of vegetables and fruit which are high in water content, and will add to this consumption.

There are many different ways of consuming water. Pleasant drinks can be made by squeezing whole fruits or vegetables. In this way we can ingest more vitamins and it is also free from pollutants. Soft drinks that contain sugar or artificial sweeteners and sometimes caffeine type stimulants are not recommended; there is nothing in them nutritionally and should be avoided. There are many herbal teas available nowadays. They are usually free of caffeine or other stimulants and do not need milk and sugar to enhance their taste.

FIBRE

Excellent sources of fibre are in plentiful supply all the year round. Rice, bread and cereals. Unrefined plant foods – root and green vegetables, peas, beans, pulses and fruit all add to dietary fibre.

The body cannot digest or absorb fibre, it passes right through the digestive system, pushing waste products on its way through the system. At the same time it absorbs waste fluids, food residues and provides bulk in the stools. Daily consumption of fibre should be around 30 grams. This will ensure that your bodily functions will remain healthy and in good working order.

Making up a diet that is high in fibre is not difficult. Remember that fresh fruits, green and root vegetables have a high water content as well as being high in dietary fibre. On the other hand, these high fibre foods do not contain concentrated fats, sugars or salt, and they do tend to be filling without fattening, and are highly nutritious. To increase your fibre intake here are some rules to follow:

Cook potatoes baked in their jackets. It is recommended that we eat the skin of baked potatoes for the added fibre. Try to buy organic potatoes, they are usually available in most supermarkets and are labeled as being organic. (Unfortunately non-organic growers spray their crops to prevent infestation and rot. To remove chemical sprays from the skin of potatoes, first wash them in clean water into which is added two tablespoons of vinegar.)

Use wholemeal bread when making sandwiches. Eat wholemeal rolls and resist using butter on them. Toasted wholemeal bread is quite agreeable with a thin spread of low fat margarine or on its own without any fat at all.

When baking, use wholemeal flour in all your recipes. (When substituting wholemeal flour for white flour always remember to add extra fluid to make up for the extra fibre in the flour.)

As a side dish or as a main meal, make up a salad to include shredded or grated raw vegetables. Instead of using salad creams, use a vinaigrette to add taste and zest to your salad.

SALT

Salt is made up of 60% *chloride* and 40% *sodium*. It is the *sodium* in salt which performs an important role in regulating the fluid balance in our bodies. Salt is also necessary to ensure that our muscles and nerves work properly and to help us maintain normal blood pressure. The amount of *sodium* that we actually need in our diet is estimated to be just over 1.5 grams per day. We easily consume this amount each day from the *sodium* which occurs naturally in our food, so it is unnecessary to add salt when cooking.

Foods With A High Salt Content

Table Salt	Salted Butter	Smoked Fish
Bread Tomato	Ketchup	Canned Soup
Baked Beans	Sausages	Breakfast Cereals
Pickles	Milk	Salad Dressings
Dry Roasted Nuts	Salad Dressings	Salted Peanuts
Cured Meat	Very Low Fat Spreads	Tinned Meat
Crisps	Shellfish	Stock Cubes
Fish Fingers	Bacon	Hard Cheese

Avoid using stock cubes, gravy granules and commercially prepared sauces for cooking. Use instead your own stock by using the juices from cooked vegetables. Use herbs and spices in your cooking. Lemon juice will also enhance the natural flavour of food.

FOODS TO AVOID

All food gives energy, of one kind or another. But there are foods that actually slow you down.

'Comfort foods' are generally sweet foods that fill you temporarily but leave you ravenously hungry in a short time. They can also be rich in high-calorie fats. A diet for 'increased' energy removes as much of this type of food from the diet as possible.

Most comfort foods are highly processed and can cause problems. White bread, instant mashed potato and other heavily processed foods pack the body with refined starch and are frequently low in minerals, vitamins, fibre and protein, they should all be avoided. Other comfort foods you should try to avoid include pastries and biscuits.

Try to avoid processed meat products, like pies and sausages. These are very fatty and contain many more calories than the fresh made varieties. If you make your own, try to use lean meat and make the pastry with margarine.

When you shop for sausages, choose varieties with a high meat content. Legally, pork sausages need contain only 65% meat, which means the rest might be made with all kinds of very fattening substances.

Instead of refined white sugar use honey or raw brown sugar. The latter contains more minerals and is more beneficial for you.

For cooking, use a strong mature Cheddar cheese. You will need less of it to flavour your food than most milder cheeses.

All fats – butter, vegetable oils, margarine – are fattening. So keep a check on everything you use in your food, including fats used in the cooking process.

Look for low-fat margarines and spreads that are high in polyunsaturates. Those that aren't might contain more fat than you would expect.

If you must snack, choose fresh fruit or vegetables rather than biscuits or sweets.

Look for low-fat varieties of your favourite foods. This includes semi-skimmed or skimmed milk, low-fat yoghurt, low-fat sausages and crisps. But remember to watch the small print, since some are much higher in calories than other reduced-calorie products.

Remember the words 'light' and 'lite' on labels do not always refer to calorie content. They might mean colour, taste or alcoholic strength and might actually be higher in calories than similar products without the 'light/lite' reference.

Cut out mayonnaise. Just a tiny amount contains lots of calories and most people are not satisfied with a tiny amount. So they pile on lots and suffer the consequences.

Cut down on saturated or hard animal fats found in butter, cheese, meat, lard or suet.

Here is a short list of comfort foods for you to avoid:

Beer
Biscuits
White bread
Cakes
Full fruit yoghurts
Marmalade
Processed meats
salted nuts
Patés
Pies and tarts
Ice cream
Instant mashed potato
Chocolates
Cream cheese
Salami

Potato chips
Cream
Crisps
Croissants
Tinned fruit in syrup
Sausages
Soft drinks
Sweets
Jam
Treacle or syrup
Soups with added cream
Tinned meats
Sugar

EATING OUT

Be mindful when eating out. If you have invited friends, let them know beforehand that your eating patterns have changed. When dining at restaurants select low-calorie foods from the menu.

If you weaken your resolve and yield to temptation, don't consider yourself a failure. Go back to the basic programme and gradually you will persevere in your endeavour on 'The Clean Liver Cleansing Programme'. When you do reach your target, be mindful that it is often just as much a challenge to continue the good that you have accomplished. It is therefore important to have the right attitude, and to establish a lifetime plan that will maintain optimum good health for many years to come.

COOKING TIPS

Cut down on fat by part-cooking food in a microwave. Sausages and chops can be partially cooked in the microwave first to remove a lot of the fat and then browned in a nonstick pan or under the grill.

Always use nonstick frying pans to cut down on the amount of fat needed for cooking.

Choose lean cuts of meat and trim off all visible fat and skin.

Chicken and turkey are only low in calories if the skin is removed. Most of the calories are contained in the skin (including fat needed to cook it) and the immediate next layer.

If you use butter or margarine on bread, soften it first so you won't use so much.

WHEN YOU SHOULD NEVER EAT

If you don't feel hungry, don't eat. How many times a day are we tempted by the sounds and smells of food. Go into any supermarket and immediately our senses are attacked with the artificial aroma of bread and cakes being baked. On the way out past the checkout we see the restaurant, beckoning with the aromatic aroma of coffee wafting close by the exit. Ignore these traps, you know it makes sense.

Never eat when you feel stressed or anxious. At times of stress your blood flow is diverted away from the liver and stomach to other parts of the body. Eating at this time will lead to bloating of the stomach and consequently poor digestion.

Never eat before lying down to rest. When you lie down to rest your body metabolism gradually slows down. In turn your stomach will empty more slowly which will encourage regurgitation and heartburn.

Never eat just before taking strenuous exercise. When you have eaten a large meal more blood is diverted to the *stomach* to aid in the digestion of your meal. Strenuous exercise immediately after a meal can cause your food to regurgitate with stomach acid coming up into the *oesophagus.* (Weight-trainers usually have a meal high in carbohydrates 2 to 3 hours before training, or when entering contests. This allows them to 'pump' up their muscles to show them off to the best of their capacity.)

Never eat before having a blood test. Some hospitals and clinics now require patients to fast for 6 hours before taking blood for certain types of blood test. This helps the hæmatologist to make a more accurate assessment of the blood samples received.

Never eat before a surgical operation. Many patients are prone to feeling sick after an operation, due to the application of an anæsthetic. Fasting for several hours is a precaution by the anæsthetist to prevent vomiting, and also to empty the stomach and bowel.

CARBOHYDRATES

Starches are your best source of carbohydrates, each gram providing approximately 4 calories. Carbohydrates are broken down by the body to produce glucose. Excess carbohydrates are stored in the liver and muscles in the form of glycogen until it is needed by the body. If we overeat on carbohydrates then the excessive glycogen will be converted to fat. Foods that include this valuable source of energy are cereals, potatoes, some root varieties of vegetables, bread, rice, oats and other grains, beans and peas. Avoid simple carbohydrates such as refined sugars and other highly processed foods that contain sugar.

Chapter 3

The Complete Liver Cleansing Programme

PLEASE STUDY THIS PROGRAMME. IT IS YOUR GUIDE TO GOOD HEALTH

In case of a serious illness involving viruses, fatigue and intake of STRONG DRUGS, ANTIBIOTICS, VACCINATIONS and ANAESTHETICS, suspend the programme until you have recovered.

DETOXIFICATION OF THE LIVER

> Start the detoxification programme on a weekend or a period of time when you will be fairly inactive.

It is essential that the liver should be detoxified before embarking on a process of improving your digestion. The liver plays a major part in the purification processes of our body and it determines which substances are to be eliminated from the body, which are to be stored, converted or produced. Particular attention should be given to the liver on a detoxification programme, as it is the liver's task during a 'fast' to clean out all the toxins remaining in all the organs and particularly in the blood.

For the first two days of your programme it will be necessary to carry out procedures to detoxify your liver of poisons and impurities. The procedure is as follows:

Fast for the first day, refresh yourself with numerous glasses of sparkling mineral water with the juice of half a lemon squeezed into each.

On the second day continue to drink plenty of water and in addition you may drink the following soup to aid your digestion. Make sufficient soup to fill two soup bowls. Drink one bowl at midday and one at 6 p.m.

- Place a selection of green vegetables into a food processor with the addition of carrots, peppers, tomatoes, plenty of seasoning and the juice of one lemon and a little water. Chop well. Place the chopped vegetables in a saucepan and bring to the boil. Allow the soup to simmer for five minutes.

DO NOT SEASON YOUR SOUP WITH SALT AS IT CAN CAUSE WATER RETENTION.

Green leafy vegetables contain plenty of chlorophyll which will dispel bad air, they also have a mild laxative and diuretic effect, consequently purifying the whole system.

> In Chinese medicine, diet is considered to be a very important part of the overall balance of the health and well-being of the body. If an individual follows a healthy, well-balanced diet, then the body will remain healthy and strong enough to fight infections.

To continue with the detoxification programme it is desirable that a period of a further three days should be given to bringing your liver into accord with your new diet. THIS CANNOT BE HURRIED. All radical changes to diet and way of life need to be gradual.

The following three day plan has been carefully chosen to bring your liver back to full working capacity under the new management of a good, healthy diet.

Day One

Breakfast	2	medium sized apples, peeled and chopped
	1	tablespoon of chopped mixed nuts
	1	teaspoon of honey
		juice of half an orange
	2	tablespoons of low fat bio-yoghurt
	Make a dressing with the yoghurt, orange juice and honey. Place the fruit and nuts in a bowl and pour the dressing over the top.	
Lunch	1	serving of baked apple, stuffed with currants and sultanas and chopped mixed nuts
	1	cup of dandelion tea
Main Meal	2	large apples, peeled and sliced
	1	hard boiled egg, with the yolk discarded
	1	teaspoon of honey
		juice of half an orange
	1	tablespoon of chopped mixed nuts
	1	medium sized beetroot, cooked peeled and sliced
	Make a dressing with the yoghurt, orange juice and honey. Place the fruit, egg, beetroot and nuts in a bowl and pour the dressing over the top.	

Day Two

Breakfast	1	glass of fresh orange juice
	1	boiled egg with the yolk discarded
	1	cup of tea or coffee with milk
Lunch	2	low calorie crispbreads, spread with low fat spread and a thin slice of Gouda cheese
	1	cup of dandelion tea
Main Meal	1	bowl of vegetable soup
	1	portion of steamed white fish, served with a mixed salad which includes dandelion leaves
	1	cup of tea or coffee with milk

Day Three

Breakfast	1	wine glass of apple juice
	1	slice of toasted wholemeal bread with grilled tomatoes or grilled mushrooms
	1	cup of tea or coffee with milk
Lunch	1	small carton of low fat bio-yoghurt
	2	sticks of celery
	1	dessertspoon of sultanas
	2	dates, chopped
	Mix all ingredients together and pour yoghurt over the top.	
	1	cup of dandelion tea
Main Meal	1	medium size portion of smoked or fresh haddock, served with a wedge of lemon
	2	tablespoons of fresh cooked spinach
	1	glass of apple juice

Continue to drink plenty of water or fruit and vegetable juices throughout the three days.

WEIGHT PROBLEMS

WARNING: A rapid weight loss could cause fatigue and an imbalance.

Losing weight too fast is not a healthy thing to do. If you find that you have lost too much weight during the past five days. Then what you need is a high energy diet to quickly build up your stamina without overloading your body

Important rules to keep your energy level high

1. Don't ever fill yourself up
2. Eat lots of raw fruits and vegetables
3. Don't eat highly processed foods packed with chemical additives

The following foods are high in energy giving minerals and vitamins:

Apples	Bread, wholemeal
Bananas	Crispbreads
Peaches, raw	Rice, brown or white
Pears, raw	Spaghetti, white or wholemeal
Peas, split	Macaroni, white or wholemeal
Potatoes	Pasta, white or wholemeal
Swedes	Porridge oats, cooked or uncooked
Sweetcorn	Lentils, all kinds
Carrots	Beans, dried
Milk	Beetroot
Yoghurt	Parsnips

For a really good start to the day, try taking the following energy shake.

8 fl oz plain yoghurt
A handful of strawberries or raspberries
1 teaspoon honey or blackstrap molasses
1 tablespoon of coconut
A squeeze of lemon juice

Combine the ingredients in a blender or food processor. Drink a large glassful first thing in the morning.

STARVING IS NOT HELPFUL AND OVEREATING CAN CAUSE HEALTH PROBLEMS

WHAT *IS* IMPORTANT IS: The QUANTITY of what you eat – not in calories but in VOLUME! Eat everything, but in small quantities and learn how to vary your food.

A GOOD NIGHT'S SLEEP IS NECESSARY: You should sleep well, soundly, without nightmares, without interruptions and you should not feel tired when you wake up in the morning.

THE WAY FORWARD

When you return to your normal diet it is a good idea to cleanse the liver in a safe and controlled manner periodically. It is advocated that it should be cleansed of its toxins by ingesting only pure fruit and vegetable juices for one day a fortnight, or if this is too severe then one day a month. Fresh fruit and vegetable juices are full of vitamins and minerals in a readily digestible form, which means they nourish as they cleanse. For beginners this may be difficult to keep to, but with perseverance you will be rewarded with increased good health, improved vitality, and you may also lose some unwanted body fat.

A one day detoxification means abstaining from your normal diet for twenty four hours not twelve. It is recommended that you abstain from first thing in the morning until the same time next day, however the period you choose is up to you. Choose a day when there are few demands on your time and energy.

It is difficult to do without food when you have to work. Or have relatives or visitors to attend to. Begin the day before by eating plain wholefoods; cooked and raw vegetables and salads. Try to avoid animal products and sweetened foods, drink fruit juice, water and herbal teas in place of coffee, tea and alcohol.

Whilst on your diet you can drink fruit and vegetable juices. It is not advisable to mix them together in the same glass or they tend to cause flatulence. Carrot and apple juice is the exception. Unlimited amounts of spring water or filtered water and non-carbonated water are all permitted.

Ending your detoxification programme correctly is as important as the preparation. Fueled by hunger pains you may be tempted to overeat on the first day. To do so would render the whole process a waste of time. So gradually wean yourself back onto solid foods, starting with small amounts of vegetables, fruit and salads and vegetable soups. You can then start eating moderately, the other foods that you have chosen for your balanced diet.

Most fruits and vegetables can be juiced and it is a good idea to include different types for flavour and the particular nutrients and properties they possess.

Suggested Herbs, Fruits And Vegetables To Calm and Cleanse Your Liver

Watermelon is an excellent diuretic; apples contain numerous vitamins and a substance called pectin which helps to remove toxins. Vegetable juices such as carrot, spinach, beetroot, celery and tomato can combine to make delicious aperitifs. Season vegetable juices with herbs if you like, but do not add salt as this can cause water retention. Oatstraw, red clover and alfalfa all calm the liver and ginseng, codonopsis and astragalus root will serve your liver as a tonic.

Chapter 4

The Balanced Diet For Health

YOU MUST HEED THE FOLLOWING RECOMMENDATIONS CONSCIENTIOUSLY:

- ☐ You can eat some wholemeal bread for breakfast but not for lunch or dinner.
- ☐ You may have a teaspoon of honey with breakfast.
- ☐ Don't eat too much fruit: two pieces a day is sufficient.
- ☐ Rice, potatoes and pasta are acceptable in normal amounts.
- ☐ Sweet drinks: avoid carbonated drinks totally.
- ☐ It is VERY IMPORTANT for your body's mineral balance to eat a little bit of everything in moderation.
- ☐ Try to avoid drinking more than 2 cups of coffee or tea daily.

CORRECT NUTRITION

Correct nutrition is important while on The Balanced Diet for Health.

- □ Do not change your new lifestyle during the diet.
- □ Do not take any new medications during the diet.
- □ DO NOT CHANGE ANYTHING until the end of the diet except in extreme cases.
- □ Try to EXERCISE to help eliminate the stress in your life.

THE BALANCED DIET FOR HEALTH DEPENDS ON THESE FACTORS:

1. Each day choose one of the seven breakfasts, seven lunches and seven main meals.
2. You are permitted to drink 500 ml of skimmed milk each day for use in tea and coffee, and where referred to in menus.
3. There is no necessity to limit the intake of low calorie drinks such as water, fruit and vegetable juices.

Any time you are enticed away from The Balanced Diet for Health substitute your craving with a piece of fruit instead. This will ensure that you will continue your diet to the maximum advantage without having to start again from the beginning.

Day One

Breakfast	½	grapefruit, no sugar allowed
	1	slice wholemeal bread, toasted with grilled tomatoes
	1	cup of dandelion tea

Lunch	1	mixed salad using all kinds of fresh vegetables served with a little oil and lemon
	1	glass of fruit or vegetable juice
Main Meal	1	turkey breast slice, served with steamed carrots and peas
	1	baked apple, stuffed with currants and sultanas and chopped mixed nuts
	1	cup of tea or coffee

Day Two

Breakfast	1	glass of fresh orange juice
	1	slice of wholemeal bread, toasted with grilled mushrooms
	1	cup of tea or coffee with milk
Lunch	1	serving spaghetti with tomato sauce
	1	cup of dandelion tea
Main Meal	1	bowl of vegetable soup
	1	portion of steamed fish, served with a mixed salad which includes dandelion leaves
	1	apple

Day Three

Breakfast	1	glass of tomato juice
	1	bowl of muesli with skimmed milk
	1	banana
Lunch	1	serving of leak and potato soup
	1	low fat bio-yoghurt sprinkled with grated hazel nuts
	1	glass of fruit or vegetable juice

Main Meal	1	portion of grilled skinless chicken breast, seasoned and served with steamed broccoli, carrots and boiled mashed swede seasoned with pepper
	1	bowl of 8 stewed prunes
	1	cup of herbal tea or coffee

Day Four

Breakfast	1	glass of fresh orange
	1	bowl of shredded wheat with milk with one teaspoon of honey to sweeten
	1	cup of tea or coffee
Lunch	1	large baked jacket potato topped with fromage frais and chopped chives
	1	glass of fruit or vegetable juice
Main Meal	1	serving of steamed white fish, served with a green salad including dandelion leaves
	1	fresh peach or any seasonal fruit

Day Five

Breakfast	1	glass of fresh fruit juice
	1	slice of toasted wholemeal bread, topped with 100mg sliced mushrooms cooked in their own juice and a tablespoon of yoghurt added.
	1	cup of herbal tea, of your own choice
Lunch	1	serving of tuna and green salad
	1	bowl of fresh strawberries or fruit in season
	1	glass of fruit or vegetable juice

Main Meal	1	portion of melon or a few grapes
	1	portion of nut roast, served with broccoli and a side salad of tomatoes, celery, cucumber and dandelion leaves
	1	carton of low fat bio-yoghurt

Day Six

Breakfast	½	grapefruit
	1	bowl of branflakes with skimmed milk
	1	banana
	1	cup of herbal tea, of your own choice
Lunch	1	two eggs (with one yolk discarded) mushroom omelette
	1	glass of fruit or vegetable juice
Main Meal	1	bowl of onion soup
	1	portion of vegetable lasagne, served with mixed salad
	1	cup of black coffee or herbal tea

Day Seven

Breakfast	1	bowl of porridge, made with milk and water. Use a little salt to season or sweeten with one teaspoon of honey
	1	cup of tea or coffee
Lunch	1	mixed green salad served with a cider vinegar and olive oil dressing
	1	handful of washed raisins or grapes
	1	glass of fresh orange
Main Meal	1	grilled chicken drumstick, with the skin removed and seasoned with herbs on a bed of roast mixed vegetables
	1	glass of fruit or vegetable juice

When you have come to the end of The Balanced Diet for Health, be sure to follow the recommendations for taking control of your metabolism given in Chapter Two.

To continue with maintaining your body in top condition, be guided by the foods and recipes given in the following pages.

Breakfast

Beginning the day with breakfast is an essential part of our diet. Without it, our energy levels begin to ebb and towards mid-morning acids begin to form in the stomach. How much better it is to give the stomach something to work on so that we feel the benefit of the energy our breakfast food provides.

A good breakfast supplies at least a quarter of the daily dietary needs. Adequate protein should be accounted for, along with carbohydrates for energy, provided by fruits and grains. Protein foods tend to maintain the blood sugar above the fasting level for a longer period of time than do carbohydrates. In order to maintain the blood sugar level throughout the morning, there must be at least 15 grams of protein in the breakfast meal.

Whole-grain cereals with skimmed or semi-skimmed milk and wholemeal toast and fruit are 'healthy' options to the traditional fried breakfast, and are often preferred by the family first thing in the morning.

Suggestions are:

- Muesli with sliced banana
- Wholemeal bread

- Low fat spread
- Fruit
- Grilled tomatoes
- Melon chopped with fruit or a slice of melon on its own
- Porridge with a teaspoon of honey
- Grilled mushrooms
- Baked beans
- Poached or scrambled egg

Midday and evening meals are interchangeable, depending on whether the main meal is taken at midday followed by a light meal or snack for tea or supper, or vice versa. Suggestions for packed lunches can also double up as supper meals, or be extended further for family picnics and outings.

Lunch

Packing a lunch is a daily routine in many homes. It should not be thought of as something to tide us over until supper. It is a meal in itself and requires just as much preparation as the meal you set on the table.

A nutritionally balanced lunch will contain at least one third of the day's requirements of protein, calories, minerals, and vitamins. It should also be fitted in with the individuals nutritional needs. Here are some suggestions for persons doing different kinds of work. The amounts included will vary, depending upon the one for whom it is planned.

For The Not So Active

- Cottage cheese and lettuce sandwich on whole-wheat bread

- □ Raw carrot strips
- □ Small carton low fat yoghurt
- □ 2 oatmeal biscuits

For The Moderately Active

- □ Egg sandwich on whole-wheat bread
- □ Fruit salad or red apple
- □ 2 Wheat germ biscuits
- □ ¼ litre skimmed milk

For The Very Active

- □ 2 Whole-wheat rolls with lentil patties
- □ Nut-bread sandwich with cream cheese
- □ Potato salad
- □ Celery sticks
- □ ½ litre of milk
- □ Red apple
- □ 2 oatmeal biscuits

Main meal

Ideally the main meal should come at midday, thus replenishing energy stores for the remainder of the work day. In any families this is difficult because of work and school schedules. Since your day has already included a good breakfast and an ample lunch or dinner, your evening meal can be simple and yet round out your nutrient intake for the day. Most of the day's work is finished, so this meal need not be so large as the other two.

Menu One

- Soup of your choice
- Fresh vegetable salad
- Whole-wheat bread with low fat spread
- Tea or coffee

Menu Two

- Cottage cheese with fresh fruit
- Oatmeal bread with low fat spread
- Tea or coffee

Foods To Nibble On When Hungry

Carrot strips	Olives
Celery	Fresh fruit
Radishes	Dried fruit
Crisp lettuce	Sunflower seeds

Healthy Food Substitutes

Coffee or tea	Decaffeinated coffee or herbal tea
Sugar, including brown sugar	Honey
Croutons in salads	Sprouts, alfalfa, mung beans
Chocolate	Carob
Carbonated soft drinks	Raw fruit/vegetable juices
White flour, rice and other refined grains	Brown flour, rice, millet or other whole grains
Packaged refined cereals	organic oatmeal, muesli
Saturated cooking oil	Olive oil
Battery chicken eggs	Free range/organic eggs
Red meat	Free range/organic poultry, meat and fish
Tinned/frozen vegetables	Fresh vegetables, including raw salads
Tinned or frozen fruit	Fresh fruit
fried foods	Grilled, baked or steamed

Rice Dishes

Rice is exceptionally good, it is a high-fibre food, meaning it passes quickly through the body and makes fat retention less likely. It also keeps the blood sugar topped up and keeps hunger at bay. Rice can be used in all kinds of meals including baked vegetables and stir-fry vegetables, salads and stews.

Following are a few recipes some of which contain rice to get your diet off to a flying start.

Wild Mushroom and Pine Nut Salad

30g cooked rice
200g fresh wild mushrooms, sliced
¼ teaspoon each of fresh tarragon, fresh parsley and fresh thyme, chopped
bunch of oakleaf and radicchio leaves, enough for 2 servings
1 teaspoon toasted pine nuts
1 salad tomato, diced
2 tablespoons olive oil
1 tablespoon of balsamic vinegar
salt and ground black pepper for seasoning

Season the balsamic vinegar with salt and pepper. Add the olive oil and whisk together in a mixing bowl.

Heat the mushrooms in a pan and sauté in their own juice until softened. Add the herbs and vinaigrette to the mushrooms and stir together.

Place the hot mushrooms in a bowl with the lettuce leaves and toss together. Add the pine nuts and diced tomatoes. Serve whilst the rice is still hot.

Celeriac and Pine Nut Salad

4 to 5 lettuce leaves
1 small onion, thinly sliced
1 tablespoon pine nuts
30g red cabbage, shredded
30g celeriac, shredded into match stick lengths
1 tablespoon seedless raisins
1 tablespoon olive oil

Brown the onion slices and pine nuts under a grill until the nuts are browned evenly and the onions are crisp. Place the celeriac, red cabbage and raisins into a large bowl and mix in the onions and nuts.

Pour the olive oil over the ingredients; toss the vegetables thoroughly to mix with the dressing.

Place on a serving dish over a bed of crispy lettuce leaves.

Vegetable Medley

3 to 4 charlotte potatoes, boiled
½ carrot, sliced
½ small leek, sliced
3 small broccoli florets, sliced
1 salad tomato, cut into quarters

Place the vegetables on a serving dish with the tomato quarters on top.

Add seasoning to suit your taste.

Rice, Spinach and Nuts

30g of rice, boiled
bunch of fresh spinach leaves
1 tablespoon of walnut pieces

juice of one lemon
salt and pepper for seasoning
1 tablespoon of brown bread crumbs
parsley to season

Wash and cook the spinach. When soft, drain it in a sieve, and press out as much of the liquid as you can. Chop it finely and mix it into the rice. Add the walnut pieces and add the lemon juice and seasoning to taste. This can be served straight from the pan or put into the oven and baked with a bread-crumb topping.

Rice and Lentil Salad

30g rice, boiled
handful of brown or green lentils, boiled
1 tomato, peeled and chopped
2 to 3 spring onions, chopped
coriander to season
1 tablespoon of low fat bio-yoghurt
squeeze of lemon juice
salt and pepper for seasoning

Cook the rice and lentils separately. Drain and mix together and leave to cool. Stir in the tomatoes, chopped spring onions, coriander and the yoghurt, mix in the lemon juice. Season and serve hot or cold.

Chapter 5

Simple Inexpensive Remedies

Modern living with all its problems and worries, as well as other detrimental influences, puts a great strain on the liver, and other organs of the body. To alleviate our anxiety, it is always good to be reminded of some of the simple remedies which can be made from natural foods and herbs, that help alleviate and sometimes cure the illnesses that befall us.

Bronchitis (and chronic colds)

Bronchitis varies greatly in severity from a mere cold to a condition in which the patient has to fight for breath. It is caused by the swelling of the mucous membranes of the lungs. The earliest symptoms, as a rule, is an irritating watery flow from the eyes and nose, with frequent attacks of sneezing and a sore throat. Factors that may cause bronchitis include long-term infections, such as chronic colds which are caused by a contagious viral infection of the upper respiratory tract.

Orthodox treatment includes bed rest, cough and pain relieving drugs, and antibiotics. To reduce mucus, avoid eating dairy products and eat only wholefoods. Garlic should be eaten raw in the diet or the oil taken as a supplement. Drink plenty of fluids to remove the toxins that have built up in the liver and to prevent dehydration. Avoid dry, overheated rooms.

Cirrhosis Of The Liver

Cirrhosis results from continuing damage to the liver where there is cell death and hardened scar tissue forms. This prevents normal liver function and cuts off the healthy liver cells from the blood supply they need. Symptoms include weight loss, loss of appetite, continuous indigestion, nausea, vomiting and general malaise.

Cirrhosis is treated by slowing the liver cell damage, mainly by abstaining from alcohol. Diuretic or antibiotic drugs may be used. Treatment consists of removing any precipitating factors such as alcohol or bile obstruction, decreased salt intake, replacement therapy and general measures depending upon the original cause.

Cramps

This is a particularly painful affliction which, fortunately is of short duration, though it might re-occur.

Any muscle can be affected but most often it is the muscles of the legs and feet that are attacked. Cramp is usually brought about by exposure to cold or after extreme exertion. Night cramps usually occur when a limb is stretched although the slightest movement can bring on an attack.

Relief can be brought about by stretching the affected muscles, or by heat and massage to relieve the pain.

A decoction of crampbark can give relief. To one cup of

boiling water add 1 dessertspoon of herbs. Allow to brew for ten minutes before drinking. Take this brew 3 times a day. To improve the circulation make a decoction with 1 dessertspoon of prickly ash and ginger combined in 260ml of boiling water. Allow to brew for 10 minutes. Drink 1 cupful 3 times a day.

Constipation and how to avoid it

The most common cause of constipation is poor diet. Other causes are stress or the lack of exercise and fresh air. There are however, many cases of constipation, in which the cause cannot be found. It may be due to insufficient bile secretion from the liver; while there are persons who naturally have an underactive bowel.

Symptoms of constipation are many. These include a coated tongue, flatulence, bad taste in the mouth, headaches and irritability. More serious complications can arise from a high temperature due to toxins not being cleared from the body. The latter being a sure sign that the liver is under par and needs cleansing.

Self help remedies include adding more fibre to your diet, drinking more fluids and getting plenty of exercise. Avoid the use of laxatives. They may seem to be a good idea but they can be addictive and overuse can cause more problem than they solve.

A herbal remedy can be made by crushing 2 senna pods into a cup of boiling water and adding a small piece of liquorice root. Allow to brew for ten minutes before drinking.

Digestive problems

Scientists now say that a major cause of dyspepsia (upset stomach) is the bacterial strain, Helicobacter pylori. If you suffer from acid indigestion, take honey to relieve the pain. If the problem is chronic, take honey at bedtime on an empty stomach.

Mix one teaspoon of honey in half a cup of hot water. Drink the honey-water whilst still hot.

Bloated Abdomen

Overeating has many ways of manifesting the problems it creates. Acid stomach, sour stomach ; these are just two of the names to describe a bloated stomach. Fortunately relief is never far away as there are many medicaments available including the herbal remedies given below.

Carrot juice contains one of the essential oils that affects the mucous membranes and stimulates the blood circulation in the stomach and intestinal tissues. Beetroot juice contains betaine, which will stimulate the function of the liver cells and protects the liver and *bile ducts* in cases of disorder.

Halitosis

Bad breath is a common but embarrassing problem that can be caused by many different conditions. Chinese medical practitioners say 'the stomach is the organ of the mouth', so if we follow this line of process then it is the stomach that causes bad breath.

Bad breath can be due to poor oral hygiene, mouth or dental infections, eating certain foods such as garlic and onions, drinking alcohol or the use of tobacco. Some diseases cause odour such as acetone in diabetes and ammonia in liver disease.

There are many remedies to help restore oral freshness. An infusion of 2 teaspoons of dried herbs made with Chinese golden thread drunk 3 times a day or if preferred use it as a gargle. Herbs such as radish and celery seeds can be sprinkled over hot or cold food as a condiment. Peppermint tea is also recommended.

Headaches

Almost everyone experiences a headache at some time. Most are the result of stress or over work. Usually a pill or tablet is taken and time becomes the healer. Although a headache is not in itself a disease, it can be a symptom of some other ailment that remains untreated. A toxic or sick liver can cause a headache. Headaches caused by less serious ailments may be classified as follows:

Migraine

The cause of migraine is still mostly uncertain. The theory is that spasms of the blood vessels occur, which interfere with the blood supply to the brain which causes temporary cerebral anemia, it is then followed by an excessive flow of blood to the brain.

One of the causes may be due to the absorption of toxins from the intestines. Migraine sufferers are therefore often advised to change their diet in the hope that it will ease the suffering.

Congestive Headache

This can be brought about by overeating, abuse of alcohol or worry. Congestive headache can be distinguished from other forms by flushing of the face and throbbing in the head, or just a dull pain in the forehead.

Toxæmic Headache

This is primarily brought about by toxins being absorbed into the blood from the intestines and circulating around the body.

It is usual to blame headaches on the liver, hence the saying *'I feel liverish'*. But in most cases it is the stomach that is suffering from over indulgence of fatty, sweet food. Both toxæmic and congestive headaches are treated with plenty of fresh water to flush the system of toxins.

HEART PROBLEMS

Angina

It is usually narrowing at the origins of the large coronary arteries which produces angina. The pain usually occurs on exertion or extreme emotion, and is described as 'crushing', 'squeezing' or 'like a band'. It is never a really sharp pain. Due to the nature of the nerve supply to the heart, the pain may radiate away from the centre of the chest to the arms or shoulders (usually the left), the neck or jaw and teeth. Occasionally it radiates to the back or the upper abdomen. In the latter case it may be confused with indigestion and correct treatment may be delayed.

Atherosclerosis

This a common disorder of the arteries. Plaques of cholesterol, fats and other residue are deposited in the walls of large and medium-sized arteries. The vessel walls become hardened and thick and the vessel narrows. This decreases circulation to organs and other regions normally supplied by the artery. It is not clear how atherosclerosis develops. It may begin with an increase of muscle in the vessel walls or by injury. Other causes may be excessive saturated fats in the diet which the liver is unable to cope with, faulty carbohydrate processing, or a genetic defect. Atherosclerosis usually occurs with ageing. It is often linked to overweight, high blood pressure, and diabetes.

Sufferers from this disease should consider radically changing their diet to a more healthy one. Garlic should be taken daily either in capsule form or eaten in the diet. Increase the amount of dietary fibre by eating more fruit and vegetables and cut out animal fats which overload the body with cholesterol.

HEPATITIS

Hepatitis is the inflammation of the liver, and the initial symptoms include a general feeling of malaise, nausea, headaches, fever and some abdominal pains. After a couple of weeks, jaundice, which is a symptom of many liver disorders, may appear involving the yellowing of eyes and skin, darkened urine and light coloured bowel movements.

Treatment of chronic hepatitis is constitutional and needs

a skilled practitioner. In cases of brief, acute hepatitis, the following remedies may be useful.

Bryonia when symptoms come on after exposure to cold and there is pain and tenderness in the liver region. Mercurius when the tongue is yellow and dirty and there is a tender liver. Phosphorus when there is a empty feeling in the abdomen and a craving for cold water followed by vomiting. Lachesis when the liver feels swollen and tender and there is a distended abdomen which is painful. Hydrastis for a swollen, tender liver with yellowish discharge from the nose and throat.

Hepatitis A (epidemic hepatitis)

This disease is transmitted by food or drink contaminated by a carrier or patient and commonly occurs where sanitation is poor. The patient becomes feverish and sick about 40 days after the incubation period. There is a yellow discoloration of the skin which appears about a week later, and persists for up to 3 weeks. Throughout the whole period the patient is highly infectious.

Hepatitis B

This disease was formerly known as serum hepatitis. It is transmitted by infected blood or blood products, contaminating hypodermic needles, blood transfusions, tattooing needles or by sexual contact.

Symptoms develop rapidly after an incubation period of 1 to 6 months. These include headaches, fever, chills, general weakness and jaundice. Recovery is gradual.

HIGH BLOOD PRESSURE (HYPERTENSION)

It is possible to tell how hard your heart is working by taking your blood pressure. The reading that you get will of course depend on several factors as blood pressure readings change slightly throughout the day, and it also depends on your level of exertion at the time it is read. It is generally considered that a reading of 120/80 is normal.

Blood pressure increases as we get older, mainly because the veins become more inflexible and do not expand so well. It is a common disorder, quite often there are no symptoms. It is characterised by high blood pressure persistently exceeding 140/90.

Essential hypertension is the most frequent kind of high blood pressure. Being overweight is one reason, it overtaxes the liver and increases the risk of high sodium levels in the blood and a high cholesterol level. Other known causes of hypertension include adrenal problems, over-active *thyroid* gland, certain kidney disorders and pregnancies. Patients with high blood pressure are advised to follow a low-sodium, low-saturated-fat diet, to reduce calories to control obesity, to exercise, to avoid stress, and to take adequate rest. Honey in the diet helps to calm the system. Take 1 teaspoon in warm water before retiring. Stop smoking tobacco and cut down on drinking tea and coffee.

HIGH CHOLESTEROL

Cholesterol is a substance found in animal fats and animal products such as egg yolks and oils. It is most common in brain tissue, *kidneys,* liver, *adrenal glands*, the blood, and fatty covers around nerve fibres. It is also manufactured by the liver in the human body to help absorb and move fatty acids. Cholesterol is needed for making numerous hormones, including the sex hormones, and for making vitamin D on the skin surface. Sometimes cholesterol hardens in the gall bladder and forms gallstones.

High levels of cholesterol in the blood are thought to be linked to the development of cholesterol deposits in the arteries and blood vessels.

Many people with high cholesterol levels are advised by their physicians to take drugs to increase *High Density Lipoprotein* cholesterol levels which may be the key to better heart and arterial health.

Sources of *High Density Lipoproteins* cholesterol can be obtained from foods such as: garlic, omega 3 oil, known as 'fish oil'. Foods rich in starch are another source. These are known nowadays as complex carbohydrates.

HOT FLUSHES AND EXCESS BODY HEAT

Hot flushes are just one of the symptoms that mostly occur in women during the menopause who approach this time with dread. There is a lot of difference in the degree of distress that this condition causes. A common symptom of excess body heat is due to an overworked or toxic liver. Herbal formulas to treat flushes and sweating work well for some people. They are usually based on *progesterone* and *oestrogen* promoting herbs. Quite a high dose of medication may be needed to begin with, and then reduced later as the condition begins to clear.

An effective herbal remedy is oil of sage; 2 to 3 drops should be added to a cup of warm water and sipped throughout the day.

Relief may also be obtained by drinking liquid sarsaparilla or ginseng tea which is very effective.

It is helpful if you can wear layers of thin clothing, so that when the hot flushes and sweating occur you can peel off an outer layer of clothing to cool yourself. Another simple method of cooling is to run cold water over your wrists, which actually works wonders.

IMMUNE SYSTEM (GENERAL INFECTIONS & WEAKNESS OF)

The immune system protects the body from invasion by making local barriers and inflammation. The main organs of the immune response system are the bone marrow, the thymus, and the lymphoid tissues. The system uses other organs too, such as the lymph nodes, the spleen, and the lymphatic vessels. The response may start as soon as the antigen invades or start as long as 48 hours later.

If the liver is not working efficiently and is unable to cleanse the blood of toxins, viruses and chemicals effectively, then the immune system will be under pressure and will not be able to combat external antigens attacking the body. Problems such as skin rashes, hives, asthma and allergies will begin to manifest themselves. It is therefore of the utmost importance to cleanse and improve the function of the *liver* by maintaining a healthy diet at all times. There are a number of alternative therapies of boosting your immune system as well as improving your diet. Additions such as vitamins and minerals in the form of capsules and tablets will add greatly to strengthening the body's defences. Dandelion tea is a very good diuretic and will help to cleanse the system.

IRRITABLE BOWEL SYNDROME

The level of discomfort that is experienced by IBS sufferers will vary from person to person, and to a lesser degree, from occasion to occasion.

In its mildest forms, Irritable Bowel Syndrome can occur as little more than frequent involuntary flatulence or belching, with the occasional period of constipation or diarrhoea.

At its worst, IBS can be crippling, with strong and repeated stomach cramps and headaches, and the inability to eat anything without immediately having to hasten to the toilet.

The vast majority of cases of IBS fall between the two extremes, and it is highly unlikely that you will fall into the extremely severe category and not have already sought medical advice.

Irritable Bowel Syndrome is an extremely aggravating disease to have to suffer from. There are several things that you can do to help yourself with this problem. There are many herbs and spices which have a pacifying effect on the stomach and digestive process. It is well worth working these into your daily diet as food additives, garnishes or herbal teas.

Dill, clove, marjoram and rosemary all add a pleasing flavour when used in food recipes, particularly rosemary with meats, dill with fish and cloves in hot sweets. Black pepper and parsley can be successfully added to the majority of meals as a garnish or during cooking. Aniseed, peppermint and spearmint go very well with several sweet and savoury dishes, and along with chamomile, fennel and lemon balm can often be found as herbal teas. Often, they can be discovered in combination teas, such as chamomile and peppermint, or lemon balm and fennel. All of these teas are very soothing, and make a delicious mid-morning drink. These herbs and spices will all help your digestive system to relax and function more naturally, and chamomile has been a well-known herbal remedy for many complaints for hundreds of years.

Working these herbs and spices into your everyday diet will have great benefits in relieving the symptoms of Irritable Bowel Syndrome, and further more, the effects they have will be completely natural and work without subjecting your body to stress.

There are some IBS conditions that are brought about because the sufferer has an intolerance to certain kinds of food. It is therefore worthwhile to leave out suspect foods one at a time from the diet to see if this is the case. Finally on the dietary side, there are several commercially packaged vitamins and minerals such as: vitamin B complex with extra biotin, and vitamin B_5, that can added to your diet in order to help reduce the effects of stress on your body, and so alleviate IBS. A herbal remedy recommends using peppermint and chamomile tea with a little ginger added, to be taken 2 to 3 times a day.

MYALGIC ENCEPHALOMYELITIS (CHRONIC FATIGUE SYNDROME)

ME is a condition characterised by the commencement of extreme fatigue after failing to recover fully from a virus infection. The weariness is accompanied by a range of other symptoms, including sore throat, muscle and joint pains, slight fever, swelling of the neck glands, headache, memory loss, and insomnia. The syndrome is diagnosed by ruling out other conditions and providing treatment to relieve the symptoms. Psychiatric counselling is often helpful in treating the depression that frequently accompanies the syndrome.

Herbalists offer gentle relaxants and tonics such as skullcap. It relaxes nervous tension while at the same time it renews and revives the central nervous system. Vervain is another herb that will strengthen the nervous system while relaxing tension and stress. An infusion can be made from either of these herbs. Use 2 teaspoons of dried herbs brewed in 1 large cup of boiling water, and drunk 3 times a day.

PANIC ATTACKS (HYPERVENTILATION)

Hyperventilation is a situation when the sufferer begins to take abnormally rapid breaths. When this happens the balance between oxygen being inhaled and carbon dioxide being exhaled becomes upset.

There are many causes for this situation to arise, such as heart attack, ischemia, fright, anxiety or panic.

When there is no underlying reason for having panic attacks it might well be that all that is needed is to improve your sleep patterns and relax your body. Chamomile has a sedative quality, which quietens the body, and for a good nights sleep drink chamomile tea sweetened with honey. The decoction is quite simple. Sweeten one cup of chamomile tea with one teaspoon of honey. Add a couple of fresh mint leaves to add a bit more interest to the drink, then drink before retiring. Before starting the day drink ginseng tea at breakfast.

PERSONALITY PROBLEMS

By personality doctors and health therapists mean – the consistent patterns of thought and behaviour with friends and loved ones throughout life. Some people are gregarious, others are happier when left alone. But what is happening when a person suddenly begins to change their pattern of behaviour for no reason at all. What do we do when a loved one suddenly becomes over emotional and irritable with all around them? Sometimes there are external influences that cause a person to change, but these soon become obvious in the course of time. It could be an underlying affliction of which the sufferer is totally unaware and consequently they refuse to be helped.

In Chinese philosophy the liver is the organ of anger. When anger is not dealt with properly it will build up and diminish the function of the liver. Chinese medicine cannot displace the anger and frustration. However, in all probability, acupuncture and herbal remedies can to a large extent help to stimulate the liver. In addition acupressure massage can bring benefits. Valerian and chamomile teas may help to calm and soothe.

POOR CIRCULATION

When the flow of blood is restricted it can lead to many serious problems the least of which includes chilblains and Raynaud's disease.

Sweet clover strengthens the capillaries and arnica will strengthen the circulation. An excellent tonic is horse chestnut which also improves the circulation, it can be used internally and externally. Gingko biloba leaves and the seed kernel are used to alleviate Raynaud's disease. This herb can be bought over the counter from any health food shop.

PROSTATE PROBLEMS

The prostate is a gland in men that surrounds the neck of the bladder and the urethra. It releases a substance that makes semen into a liquid. It is about the size of a chestnut, and is made up of muscular and glandular tissue. It is located in front of the rectum, through which it can be felt, especially when enlarged.

Prostatomegaly

This is a swelling of the prostate gland, usually caused by infection. The patient urgently needs to urinate frequently and has a burning sensation during urination. The orthodox treatment is with antibiotics, sitz baths, bed rest, and fluids. In traditional Chinese medicine the treatment is with plantain seed, water plantain, cinnamon bark and corktree bark. For non-cancerous enlargement of the prostate herbalists use diuretic herbs such as horsetails in cases of inflammation. An infusion of 2 teaspoons of the dried herb drunk 3 times a day is beneficial. Saw palmetto may also be used with safety. A decoction of 1 teaspoon of berries drunk 3 times a day will ease the flow of urine. Supplements of 15mg of zinc may reduce the swelling.

Traditional Chinese acupuncture practitioners claim to be able to relieve the symptoms of *prostatitis* and benign enlargement. Another oriental therapy is shiatsu which is concerned with prevention as well as treatment of illnesses. The purpose of a shiatsu treatment is to rebalance energies and promote self-healing. Each treatment is based on an assessment of the individual's symptoms and their physical and emotional condition. It is a deeply relaxing treatment but makes no extravagant claims.

Many conventional drugs are derived, or were originally derived, from plant extracts. Some of these extracts can be of undoubted benefit in some cases and a few are even accepted by conventional urologists! The 'saw palmetto,' is probably the most interesting plant for treating prostate disease. It appears naturally to produce chemicals which have an influence on the mechanism of benign enlargement of the prostate.

Prostate Cancer

Adenocarcinoma of the *prostate*, another name for cancer, is one of the commoner cancers. It is a slowly spreading cancer of the *prostate gland.* The cause is not known but is believed to be hormone-related. Although the patient may have no specific symptoms, the cancer may be detected due to bladder blockage, presence of blood in the urine, or other infection.

It has no clear connection with diet, drink, smoking or environmental factors although some recent studies have suggested that vasectomised men are more at risk. This however remains in dispute.

Social factors do not seem to have much influence on prostate cancer unlike with other cancers. The body's immunological response can, to some extent, keep the disease at bay. It is virtually unknown in men under 45 years and its incidence increases as we age. Prostate cancer often exists in elderly men without being evident or causing any symptoms and as men get older the more likely they are to have the latent disease. Scarcely any of these cancers cause any problems and men over 70 years with prostate cancer are far more likely to die with it than of it.

This may mirror a similar age related decline in the immunological response of the body. It is therefore predominantly a disease of rich, industrialised countries whose inhabitants have a high life expectancy.

PSORIASIS (AND SKIN CONDITIONS)

The rash begins with small red patches with thick, dry, silvery scales. It is caused by the body making too many skin cells. Sores may be anywhere on the body but are more prevalent on the scalp, ears, arms, and the pubic area. Sometimes there is a swelling of small joints which is part of the skin disease. Treatment includes blood cleansing herbs, hormone creams, ultraviolet light, tar soap baths, creams and shampoos. An infusion of dandelion root, red clover flowers and burdock may help the purification process. A preparation can be made from 1 teaspoon of each of the dried herbs brewed in 230ml of boiling water and drunk 3 times a day.

Fungal Skin Infections

Fungal skin infections are among the most common complaints. Anyone can get them because they are highly contagious and can cause secondary infections which are hard to eradicate. Usually they take hold in the body's moist, warm nooks and crannies and once they do, they cause itchy rashes and the skin starts to flake or crack. To help clear the condition take 3 to 4 garlic capsules daily or 1 clove of fresh garlic daily. Reduce the ingestion of all refined sugars and white flour.

Dry Skin

Dry skin is a very common problem extending from mild to severe. If you have a disposition towards dry skin, it will probably be a lifelong issue, and if ignored, it can become more serious. However there are many efficient and simple things you can do to prevent and relieve dry skin.

The herbs that Chinese doctors have used to treat skin disorders have met with considerable success. Some of those recommended include the Chinese herb ledebouriella sesloides, potentilla chinensis and clematis armandii. These herbs are grown on mainland China. They are ground up into a fine powder and combined in a certain mixture and made into a brew which is taken each day.

Diet can also help with skin diseases. Any underlying problem with the liver will allow toxins to be carried around in the blood and eventually to the skin. It is therefore essential to have a healthy liver in order to keep your skin in top condition.

RHEUMATIC DISEASE

There are more than 100 different types of arthritis all involving some disorder or inflammation of the joints and muscles. The two most common forms are rheumatoid arthritis and osteoarthritis. Most rheumatic and arthritic aches and pains come and go. Even the most persistent condition such as osteoarthritis may only be intermittent. But when aches and pains persist and orthodox treatment does not help enough, it is no wonder that a sufferer will try some less orthodox form of treatment. Many of our stock remedies go back hundreds of years and are part of medicine folklore.

There are many ways in which you can help yourself if you suffer from either form of rheumatic disease. Try to keep yourself mobile. Do special exercises for individual joints, these can be very helpful. Try to move your joints throughout their full range, and take care not to ignore those joints that are not affected. Do not over tax your joints, but try to keep up a full and active life as possible.

Herbal remedies are very popular and usually non-toxic. Devils claw is claimed to have given good results. It contains several glycosides that are powerful anti-inflammatory agents. A preparation can be made from 1 teaspoon of dried herbs in 1 cup of boiling water and drunk 3 times a day.

URINARY INFECTIONS

Problems affecting the *kidneys*, especially if it is an inability to pass water, are a matter for professional advice. The remedies given below are given purely to bring comfort and relief if you are feeling sluggish and low with that unpleasant feeling that your body needs a good clean out.

Herbalists recommend that you drink a brew of dandelion tea to help cleanse the system. Eat plenty of watercress, runner beans and grapes; these are all full of minerals that the body needs. Fresh water also helps to cleanse the *kidneys* as well as the liver. In addition to drinking water, eat plenty of vegetables and fruit which are high in water content, and will add to this consumption. Barley water is particularly useful to cleanse the system.

CANDIDIASIS

There are many common diseases, such as diaper rash, thrush, vaginitis, and dermatitis, they are all caused by candida infestations. A warm, moist environment will promote the growth of Candida. Some drugs will destroy beneficial bacteria as well as harmful ones and allow the fungus to grow.

Gentian violet is a drug used on the skin. Antifungal drugs, such as clotrimazole, candicidin, or nystatin may be used for some infections. Sufferers should avoid sugar and dairy products. A Chinese treatment involves drying up the damp with pinellia tuber, poria, magnolia bark and kapok flower.

Chapter 6

How To Improve Your Liver Function

LIVER TONIC

The dandelion plant has been the subject of many medical papers and has been well documented over many centuries. It may be used to treat cases where the liver is congested or inflamed, such as congestive jaundice. It can also be used as part of the treatment for muscular rheumatism. It is a powerful diuretic and is one of the best natural sources of *potassium.* This makes it an ideal well-balanced diuretic that is safe and easy to use.

The tonic is made from 2 teaspoons of the root and drunk 3 times a day. The leaves may be eaten raw in salads.

Dandelion and burdock combined make an excellent tonic. The taste is somewhat similar to beer, which may please some readers.

INTERNAL TRACT HYGIENE

Psyllium seed is obtained from the Indian plant *plantago ovata.* It dissolves or swells in the intestinal fluids and stimulates the bowels acting as a purgative. A solution of magnesium causes the retention of water in the intestine and thus also acts as a bulk-forming laxative, as does lubricant laxatives and water enemas. Saline agents in purgative doses are used in cases of food and drug poisoning. Stimulant laxatives, or enemas are frequently used prior to surgery or X-ray examination.

RID YOUR FOOD OF PESTICIDES

Over 90% of our foods have been contaminated with pesticides in one way or the other. Vegetables, fruits and cereals are sprayed as a matter of routine with one or more pesticides during the growing season, whether its needed or not.

One way of avoiding pesticides is to grow our own fruit and vegetables. For town and city folk this may not be a feasible proposition. Their only alternative is to buy organically grown food. Many supermarkets do stock a small amount of organic foods and these are labeled as such.

There is one such kitchen food that is found in almost every home and that is vinegar. Vinegar is an acidic liquid, a product obtained from the fermentation of alcohol. It is used as a condiment, preservative, cleanser and medicament. When preparing fruit and vegetables always leave them for 10 minutes or so in a bowl immersed in water to which is added two or three tablespoons of vinegar. Wash the produce again before cooking or eating to remove the taste of the vinegar.

TEAS TO PURIFY YOUR BLOOD

The purpose of herbal teas is only relevant to those who want to cleanse their body's of impurities to enable them to lead a more healthy and active life. Most have differing effects due to the variety of vitamins and minerals contained in them which are all necessary for our bodily functions.

Most supermarkets stock small packs of sachets so that each tea can be sampled before deciding which one you like the best. Many of these teas are based on chamomile, peppermint, fennel or rosehips. They are usually free of caffeine or other stimulants and do not need milk and sugar to enhance their taste.

Infusion

Should you decide to prepare the herbs yourself, the usual formula is 1 to 2 dessertspoon of herbs steeped in two cups of boiling water. Allow the herbs to brew for ten minutes before drinking. Usually the tea is drunk whilst warm or in hot weather it can be chilled, but in the case of colds or coughs, it should be taken hot. Herbal teas are mainly taken in regular small doses, and a daily intake can be between one and four cups. Sachets of tea bought over the counter in shops should be used according to the instruction given by the manufacturer.

Decoction

With this method the berries, seeds, roots and twigs are used. The formula is 28 grams of herbs to one cup of cold water. The water and herbs are placed in a pan and brought to the boil and then simmered for 20 minutes. Strain the liquid into the cup before drinking.

Valerian To Reduce Hunger and as a Relaxant

Drink as an aperitif ½ hour before meals.

Chamomile Is An All Healing Tea

Drink after meals or simply to refresh oneself.

Dandelion As a Diuretic and Cleanser

Drink as a tonic. Add a little honey to sweeten the taste.

Peppermint For The Digestion

Drink 3 times a day for relief. Peppermint tea can be sweetened with a teaspoon of honey.

Rosemary To Soothe Sore Throats

Drink 3 times a day for relief.

Sage To Soothe Stress & Shock

Sweeten with honey if desired.

Thyme For Nervous Headaches, Coughs, Colds & Depression

Drink 3 times a day for relief.

VITAMINS AND MINERALS

Vitamins and minerals are the nutrients that our body needs in very small amounts each and every day of our lives. However, despite the small amount required we need quite a range of vitamins and minerals for our good health. Some of these make up a significant proportion of the body's structure, tissues and fluids to keep them functioning normally and to carry out all the processes necessary for life.

Vitamins & Their Beneficial Effects	**Sources**	
	Herbs	**Foods**
Vitamin A (Retinol), RDA: 0.75 mg counteracts night blindness, builds resistance to respiratory infections, promotes growth of teeth, bones and hair	alfalfa, oatstraw, dock	carrots, asparagus, cayenne pepper, sorrel, carrots, kale, spinach, cress, sweet potatoes, parsley, apples, garlic, ginger, papaya, rye, peaches, nectarines, dried apricots
Vitamin B1 (Thiamin, Aneurin), RDA: 1.3 mg promotes growth, aids digestion, improves mental attitude, helps nervous system and prevents stress	oatstraw, red clover, alfalfa	rice, bran, wheatgerm, sunflower seeds, apples, garlic, papaya, turnips, rye, peanuts, oatmeal, sesame seeds
Vitamin B2, (Riboflavin, lactoflavin, Vitamin G), RDA: 1.6 mg aids growth and reproduction, promotes hair, skin and nail growth, helps eyesight	alfalfa, oatstraw, red clover	hot red chillies, wheatgerm, millet, apples, garlic, ginger, rye, leafy green vegetables, fish, eggs, yeast, cheese, liver, kidney, almonds

Vitamins & Their Beneficial Effects	Sources	
	Herbs	**Foods**
Vitamin B3 (Niacin, Nicotinic acid), RDA: 1.8 mg essential for sex hormones, increases energy, aids nervous system, helps digestion and prevents migraines	alfalfa, red clover	apples, garlic, ginger, onions, papaya, rye, turnips, wheat, parsley, watercress
Vitamin B5 (Pantothenic acid), RDA: 4-7 mg aids in healing wounds, fights infection, strengthens immune system, builds cells	barberry	rye, turnips, garlic, papaya, parsley, beans, egg yolk, legumes, liver, oranges, peanuts, wheat germ, whole-grain cereals
Vitamin B6 (Pyridoxine) RDA: 1.5-2 mg, produces anti-bodies, red blood cell formation; metabolism of protein		green vegetables, brewer's yeast, yeast extracts, fish, pulses, prunes, raisins, soya beans, flour, nuts, whole-grain cereals, milk

Vitamins & Their Beneficial Effects	Sources	
	Herbs	Foods
Vitamin B9 (Folic acid, foliate, Vitamin Bc, pteroylglutamic acid) RDA: 0.3 mg, proper functioning of vitamin B12; formation of red blood cells, use of proteins, fats and carbohydrates		liver, kidney, meat; green vegetables, fresh fruit, brewers yeast, yeast extract, wheatgerm, pulses
Vitamin B12 (Cobalamin), RDA: 2 micrograms, proper functioning of folic acid, forms and regenerates red blood cells, increases energy, improves, concentration, maintains nervous system	alfalfa, comfrey, red clover	rye, sprouted seeds, legumes, eggs, kidney, liver, milk, fish
Vitamin B17 (Amygdalin), purported to control cancer		apricots, peach seeds, apples, cherries, plums, nectarines

Vitamins & Their Beneficial Effects	Sources	
	Herbs	**Foods**
Vitamin C (Ascorbic acid), RDA: 30 mg, helps body to absorb calcium, helps form collagen, heals wounds, aids immune system		citrus fruits, apples, watercress, garlic, onions, turnips, cayenne, sweet red pepper, parsley, walnuts, lemons, green leafy vegetables, potatoes, salad vegetables, blackcurrants, rose hips
Vitamin D, (Cholecalciferol) RDA: 10 micrograms, prevents rickets, essential for calcium and phosphorus utilisation, and necessary for strong teeth and bones	alfalfa, fenugreek	apples, watercress, fish liver oils, tuna, milk, salmon, herring, mackerel, sprouted seeds
Vitamin E (Tocopherol), RDA: 10 micrograms, antioxidant, anti-coagulant, anti-ageing, possibly fertility	alfalfa, flaxseed	apples, parsley, rye, wheatgerm, whole-wheat, broccoli, eggs, green vegetables, nuts, seeds, pulses

Vitamins & Their Beneficial Effects	Sources	
	Herbs	**Foods**
Vitamin K, (Menadione), RDA: 70-140 micrograms, blood clotting		whole-grain cereals, leafy vegetables, seaweed, liver, potatoes, eggs, wheatgerm

Minerals & Their Beneficial Effects	Sources	
	Herbs	**Foods**
Calcium, RDA: 50 mg, aids blood clotting, protects and build bones and teeth, and buffers acid in the stomach	comfrey, marestail, oatstraw, liquorice	sesame seeds, seaweeds, kale, turnips, almonds, soybeans, dandelion leaves, hazelnuts, horseradish, honey, salmon
Chromium, RDA: 0.05-0.2 mg, breaks down sugar for use in the body, it deters diabetes and help maintain the correct blood pressure		wholemeal bread, potatoes, spinach, spaghetti, bananas, haddock
Copper, RDA: 0.05-0.2 mg, converts iron to haemoglobin, staves off anaemia	ephaedra	peaches, turnips

Minerals & Their Beneficial Effects	**Sources**	
	Herbs	**Foods**
Iodine, RDA: 0.14-0.15 mg, production in the thyroid gland of hormones that controls metabolism and growth and development		salt, seafood, kelp, meat, fruit, vegetables (where soils contain iodine)
Iron, RDA: 10 mg, aids growth, promotes immune system, prevents fatigue, essential for metabolism of reproduction of haemoglobin	red raspberries, yellow dock, kelp, nettle	wheat and rice, (bran and germ), brazil nuts, greens, apples, grapes, walnuts, dill, dandelion leaves, pumpkin, squash, plums
Manganese, RDA: 2.5 mg, essential for nerve and muscle functioning, known as anti stress mineral, improves cardiovascular system	comfrey, cramp bark, uva ursi, gravel root	apples, peaches, rye, turnips, tea, wholemeal bread, avocados
Molybdenum, RDA: 0.15-0.5 mg, prevention of dental caries; iron metabolism; male sexual function		buckwheat, barley, oats, liver, pulses

Minerals & Their Beneficial Effects	Sources	
	Herbs	**Foods**
Phosphorus, RDA: 800 mg, needed for formation of bones, teeth and nerve impulse transfer, assimilates niacin present in ever body cell	yeast	rice, wheat (bran and germ) squash seeds, sesame seeds, brazil nuts, fish, kale, mustard radishes, aubergine, leek, seafood
Potassium, RDA: 1875-5625 mg, regulates body's water balance, aids muscle function, helps dispose of body waste, supports allergy treatment	kelp, dulse, Irish moss	soya beans, bananas, cayenne pepper, artichokes, asparagus, cauliflower, kale, grapefruit, radishes, sorrel, tomatoes
Selenium, antioxidant, preventing or slowing down again, important for prostate glands in males, prevents skin conditions		wheatgerm, bran, onions, broccoli, tomatoes, shellfish, tuna
Sodium, RDA: 2000 mg, essential for normal growth, aids in preventing sunstroke, helps nerves and muscle function, excessive in most diets	kelp, seaweed, marigold, bladderwrack	olives, dulse, apricots, currants, figs, dates, eggs, horseradish, lentils, oats, red cabbage, strawberries, turnips, celery cayenne pepper

Minerals & Their Beneficial Effects	Sources	
	Herbs	**Foods**
Sulpher, RDA: none laid down, tones up skin and hair, helps fight bacterial infection, aids liver, part of tissue building amino acids	garlic, kelp and dandelion	onion, sprouts, coconut, cucumber, garlic, figs, egg yolk, greens, kale, okra, parsnips, potatoes, strawberries, turnips, carrots
Zinc, RDA: 15 mg, accelerates healing, prevents infertility, helps prevent prostate infections, promotes growth of teeth, bones and hair	red raspberries, alfalfa uva ursi, slippery elm	apricots, peaches, nectarines, oyster, wheatgerm, cocoa, mustard seeds, brewer's yeast eggs, pumpkin seeds

CONCLUSION

Much information has been given in this book and I hope it has been of value to you. There is so much that we can do for ourselves. With the right attitude and an intelligent outlook we can live life knowing that we have done everything possible to improve ourselves. The important thing to remember is to live life according to nature's rules.

In conclusion, when you have completed The Complete Liver Cleansing Programme, you must consider what you are going to do next. Above all, explore all new avenues with an open and realistic mind. Take control of your new self. Feel free to follow your instincts and seek to improve yourself, learn how to transcend your limitations. But, whatever decisions you make, always be mindful that it is the well-being of your body that you are striving to improve and maintain. The more you think and observe the better your body will serve and reward you.

Remember, nutrition and fitness go hand in hand, and it is important to eat foods that provide energy, and nutrients for muscular development and growth and repair of body tissues. Whatever your physical limitations, always strive to push yourself to the limit.

Bibliography

The Women's Guide To Herbal Medicine by Carol Rogers – Published by Hamish Hamilton

An Elders' Herbal by David Hoffman – Published by Healing Arts Press, Vermont, USA

Reader's Digest – Family Guide To Alternative Medicine – First Edition 1991

Traditional Chinese Medicine by Sheila Mcnamara & Dr Song Xuan Ke – Published by Hamish Hamilton, London 1995

The Prostate – A Complete Guide For The Over 40s by Martin Williams BA Msc

The Complete Family Doctor – Published by Odhams Press Ltd, England

The Nature Doctor by Dr H C A Vogel – Published in Australia by Bookman Press, 1995

Oxford Reference Concise Medical Dictionary, 1994

The New Natural Family Doctor by Gaia Books Ltd – Published in UK, 1996

Nutrition And Diet Logic by Charla Devereux – Published by Foulsham

The Natural Health Book – Published 1991 by New Burlington Books

The Hamlyn Encyclopedia Of Complementary Health – Published in Great Britain, 1996 by Hamlyn – Reed International Books Ltd

Index

Y

Z

BRISTOL HEALTH REPORTS

- How Your Liver Functions
- 100 Great Recipes

How Your Liver Functions

It is always useful to know how things work in your body. That way, when they are being discussed with your health advisor, you will at least have an idea of what is being talked about.

The liver is looked upon as the storehouse of the body and many chemical substances are dealt with and given off when the occasion arises. For example, when an increase of energy is required, the liver gets busy and manufactures energy-giving substances out of the food that has been digested, especially sugary or starchy foods. But if the diet is excessive or ill-balanced, the storage power of the liver may become over-taxed, especially if no exercise is taken to allow the liver to use up the extra sugar, etc. The liver also manufactures bile, which is an important substance in aiding digestion.

The liver is the largest gland in the body, weighing somewhere around 1200 to 1600 grams, and measuring about 30 centimetres inches from side to side and 15 centimetres at its thickest part. It is situated in the top right portion of the abdominal cavity. Dark-brown in colour and solid to the touch, its shape has some resemblance to a wedge, the thick part being towards the right and the thin part extending towards the left, and reaching several centimetres beyond the mid-line of the body. The thick part, or right lobe, as it is called, is tucked up into the right dome of the midriff, or diaphragm, and lies behind the ribs. The left lobe extends towards the middle-line of the body, and passes out from the protection of the ribs.

A large vein, called the portal vein, brings blood to the liver from the stomach and bowel, the pancreas and the spleen; and, contrary to the usual behaviour of veins, this vein breaks up into smaller veins, and these into a large capillary network which traverses the substance of the liver. Blood is also brought to the liver by the hepatic artery. Nerves of various kinds enter the organ. The hepatic duct, which is of considerable size, drains bile from the liver; this duct is joined by the cystic duct coming from the gall bladder, and then becomes the common bile duct through which bile is emptied into the duodenum, or first part of the small intestine.

The liver is made up of an immense number of lobules, circular or oval in shape, and consisting of rows of liver cells radiating from a centre which is occupied by the central or intralobular vein. Between the rows of cells are two sets of capillaries for blood and for bile, which communicate with larger vessels at the margins of the lobules. Surrounding and permeating the lobules is a delicate fibrous tissue, known as Glisson's capsule, which is continuous with the fibrous tissue investing the whole organ.

Blood flows from the periphery to the centre of a lobule, the hepatic cells meanwhile extracting from it substances for storage or excretion, and by the intralobular veins it conveys to larger veins through which it passes to the hepatic veins and is discharged into the inferior vena cava, and so reaches the heart.

Liver cells, which from mutual pressure usually assume a polygonal shape, have many activities. They produce bile, the materials for which they extract from the blood. Bilirubin, the colouring matter occurring most abundantly in human bile, though modified by its passage through a liver cell, is formed by other cells, known as Kupffer's cells, which are found in the lining of the liver-capillaries and elsewhere. Bilirubin is derived from the haemoglobin of the blood.

Liver cells also extract harmful substances from the blood, either converting them into harmless ones or excreting them in the bile. If, however, such substances are in excess in the blood, as when the digestion is out of kilter, they may not be dealt with adequately in the liver, so that a proportion passes into the blood circulating throughout the body, producing symptoms of biliousness.

Urea is formed in the liver, and is passed into the blood to be excreted by the kidneys. The liver produces fibrinogen, the substance in the blood that forms a clot, and anti-thrombin, a ferment that prevents clotting in the circulating blood, an accident that might otherwise occur owing to the death and disintegration of white blood corpuscles.

Another important function of the liver cells is to take up sugar from the blood and store it as glycogen, subsequently reconverting this into sugar to meet the demands of the body. Sugar is the fuel which supplies muscles with their energy. By the use of appropriate tests the modern clinician can measure the capacity of the liver for carrying on some of its functions.

On account of the very considerable amount of oxidation which is part of the chemical activities going on in this large gland, it is quite an important source of body heat. The liver also possesses large powers of replacing portions that are thrown out of action by disease by producing fresh cells.

100 Great Recipes to Promote Optimum Liver Function

Muesli

Ingredients:

225g rolled oats
½ cup sunflower seeds
½ cup corn or sunflower oil
Breakfast
½ cup demerara sugar
1 cup wheatgerm
Pinch of salt
½ cup mixed dried fruit
¾ cup clear honey

Mix everything but the dried fruit and sprinkle the mixture on. Spread evenly and bake in a low oven for about half an hour and stir in the dried fruit just before serving.

Egg Omelette

Ingredients:

2 eggs
1 tablespoon of water
15ml olive oil
salt and pepper for seasoning

Whisk the eggs with the water, salt and pepper. Heat the olive oil in a pan and pour in the egg mixture. Allow to cook for about half a minute when the mixture should be set on the bottom. Tilt the pan, at the same time loosening the egg mixture from the sides of the pan. Fold the omelette away from the handle and tip out onto a hot dish.

If desired, add a few cooked mushrooms, or a few slices of cooked potato to the omelette before folding.

Raspberry Yoghurt

Ingredients:

50g raspberries
125ml milk
2 teaspoons of clear honey
150g carton low fat yoghurt

This wonderful combination of tastes will refresh and set you up for the day. All that is necessary is to place the ingredients in a blender, and whisk until smooth. Sip slowly to experience a taste sensation.

Breakfast Scones

Ingredients:

250g wholemeal flour
1 teaspoon cream of tartar
1 teaspoon carbonate of soda
pinch of salt
50g margarine
125ml sour milk

Sift the dry ingredients into a bowl, rub in the margarine and make into a soft dough with the sour milk. Knead lightly then roll out to 15mm thickness and cut into rounds. Place on a floured cold baking sheet and bake in a preheated oven, 220°C (425°F, gas mark 7) for 10-15 minutes.

Honey Lemon Curd

Ingredients:

4 lemons
450g clear honey
100g butter
6 eggs (4 whole, 2 whites)

Grate the lemon rinds and squeeze the lemons. Put the juice into a double saucepan and add the butter and honey. Beat the eggs and egg yolks and fold lightly into the mixture. Cook over a gentle heat, stirring continuously until thick and creamy. Leave to cool. Pour into jars and cover.

Cream Cheese Dip

Starter.

Ingredients:

225g cream cheese
½ teaspoon ground mustard
Salt and pepper to season
2 tablespoons set honey
dash Worcestershire sauce

Beat all ingredients together, cover and chill for 2 hours. Serve with a selection of raw vegetables.

Honey Melon and Grapefruit Cocktail

Ingredients:

2 large grapefruits, peeled and cut into segments
Half a medium sized cucumber, cut into matchsticks
Half a large melon, de-seeded, skinned and cubed
1 tablespoon clear honey

Mix grapefruit cucumber and melon. Chill, Serve in individual dishes, Stir in the honey and blend together.

Florida Grapefruit

Ingredients:

2 Florida grapefruit, segmented
2 tablespoons white wine
¼ teaspoon ground nutmeg
¼ teaspoon ground cinnamon

Place the grapefruit segments and any juice in a serving bowl. Mix the wine and spices together in a non-metallic pan, and warm slightly over a low heat. Pour over the grapefruit. Cover and leave to marinate for at least 2 hours before serving.

Cinnamon Pears

Ingredients:

100ml dry cider
squeeze of lemon juice
1/2 teaspoon ground cinnamon
pinch of nutmeg
2 ripe dessert pears, peeled, cored and sliced in half
1 level teaspoon runny honey

Place the cider, spices, honey, and a squeeze of lemon juice in a pan and bring to the boil, cover and simmer for 3 minutes. Poach the pears in the cider for 20 minutes, or until soft. Serve the pears in dessert bowls with the cider marinade.

Dried Fruit Muesli

Prepare the evening beforehand.

Ingredients:

50g dried fruits, previously washed (apricots, prunes or raisins)
1 tablespoon lemon juice
2 teaspoons Barbados sugar
1 tablespoon muesli

Chop or mince the washed fruit. Add the lemon juice and sugar. Stir into the muesli. Add enough water to cover. In the morning serve with a few chopped nuts sprinkled over the top.

Fresh Fruit Muesli

Ingredients:

125g fresh fruit (apples, strawberries, raspberries, black or red currants, peaches or apricots, banana, oranges or satsumas)
2 teaspoons of Barbados sugar
2 tablespoons water
1 tablespoon basic muesli
1 tablespoon grated hazel nuts

Wash the fruit and trim. Chop, slice or mash, depending on the fruits being used. Mix in the sugar and water. Add the muesli and mix thoroughly. Sprinkle nuts over the top and serve immediately.

Porridge with Bran

Ingredients:

1 cupful of porridge oats
1 dessert spoonful bran
2 to 2½ cups of water
pinch of salt

To make super creamy porridge put the porridge oats and bran into a small saucepan and add the water. (For extra creaminess add half water and half milk.) Add salt to taste and bring to the boil. Simmer for 3 to 5 minutes, stirring occasionally.

To microwave in a 650 watt oven, place the ingredients in a non-metallic bowl. Stir and cook uncovered, on full power for 2 minutes. Remove from the oven and stir well. Replace in the oven and cook for 1 to 1½ minutes. Check that the porridge is piping hot before serving. Serve the porridge with milk for a delicious start to the day. Add a dessert spoonful of honey if a sweetener is required.

Honey Orange Pick Me Up

Ingredients:

1 cup plain non fat yoghurt
1 orange, peeled, sectioned & seeded
1 tablespoon lemon juice
½ teaspoon grated fresh orange rind
1 tablespoon honey

Process everything in blender until smooth.

Strawberry Cup

Ingredients:

5 cups strawberries
2 cups grape juice
6 tablespoons corn flour
4 tablespoons honey
¾ teaspoon lemon juice

Dissolve cornflour in juice using a wire whisk. Gently boil until clear, stirring often. Add the rest of the ingredients and cook until the strawberries are soft. Remove from heat and mash the strawberries with a potato masher. Chill in the refrigerator before using.

Plain Waffles

Ingredients:

225g wholemeal flour
½ teaspoon salt
2 eggs
150g melted margarine
2 teaspoons baking powder
250ml milk

Separate the egg yolks from the whites of the eggs. Beat the yolks with the milk. Sieve the flour, salt, and baking powder into a basin, make a well in the centre, and stir in the beaten egg yolks and milk, and the melted margarine. Beat well, and just before the waffles are ready to be cooked, fold in the stiffly beaten whites of eggs. Heat the waffle iron thoroughly, brush with oil. Pour on just enough batter to cover. Allow to rise slightly before closing the iron down tightly. Hold handles 15cm apart at the base for a few seconds. Then shut down and after 2 minutes turn the iron. Serve with warmed honey.

Kedgeree

Ingredients:

100g brown rice, cooked and drained dry
1 hard boiled egg
20g margarine
1 teaspoon of chopped parsley
125g cold cooked smoked haddock, or white fish

Chop up the white of the egg coarsely, and add to the fish, which should be flaked. Melt 20g of margarine and heat the fish in it. Add the rice, and cook a few moments longer. Pile up in an entrée dish neatly in the shape of a pyramid. Garnish with chopped parsley in a long line down the side. Sprinkle the yolk of the egg, rubbed through a sieve, over the top. Serve at once.

Mushrooms on Toast

Ingredients:

225g mushrooms
3 tablespoons milk
25g margarine
25g flour
pepper, salt and nutmeg
lemon juice
2 slices wholemeal bread, toasted

Skin and wash the mushrooms; cook very gently with 1 tablespoon of milk and the margarine in a closely covered pan for 20-30 minutes. Blend the flour with the rest of the milk, add to the mushrooms, and stir until boiling. Simmer for a few minutes longer. Season with pepper and salt, nutmeg and lemon juice. Serve the mushrooms on hot crispy toast.

Mushrooms & Onions on Toast

Ingredients:

2 slices of wholemeal bread, toasted
4 large mushrooms, washed
15g margarine
2 small onions, peeled

Chop the onions and slice the mushrooms thinly and fry these together in the margarine for 5 minutes. Put them on hot, crispy toast before serving.

Compote with Grapefruit

Ingredients:

100g mixed dried fruits, comprising prunes, apricots and peaches
225ml hot herbal tea
1 grapefruit
1 carton low fat yoghurt
1 tablespoon muesli

Place the dried fruit into a heat-proof serving bowl and pour over the hot tea. Cover with a tight fitting lid, and cook on high for 5 minutes. Leave to cool. The fruit will plump up as it cools. Cut the peel and pith away from the grapefruit with a sharp knife. Cut the fruit into segments by slicing the knife between the membranes, taking care to collect any juices. Place the segments in the serving dish with the dried fruit mixture and any juice collected while the grapefruit was being segmented. Halve or quarter any fruits that are large. Serve chilled topped with yoghurt and sprinkled with muesli.

Curried Meat Sandwich

Ingredients:

2 slices wholemeal bread
15g low calorie spread
cold meat, finely chopped; mixed with a little diced apple
1 teaspoonful of chutney
squeeze of lemon juice
1 teaspoonful curry paste
seasonings

Spread the bread with low calorie spread creamed with salt, curry paste, lemon juice and a little chutney to taste. Add the filling and cut to shape.

Chicken Sandwich

Ingredients:

2 slices wholemeal bread
15g low calorie spread
Slices of chicken breast, minced or cut very finely
several lettuce leaves, shredded
low calorie mayonnaise
seasonings

Spread the bread with low calorie spread creamed with a little salt, cayenne, and a small pinch of mustard. Add the chicken mixed with mayonnaise, add the lettuce, and cut to shape.

Egg Sandwich

Ingredients:

2 slices wholemeal bread
15g low calorie spread
several lettuce leaves, shredded
1 hard boiled egg
low calorie mayonnaise
squeeze of lemon juice
seasonings

Spread the bread with low calorie spread. Mash the egg with a little salt, lemon juice, cayenne, and mayonnaise. Add the shredded lettuce next to the egg filling and cut to shape.

Other suggestions for sandwich fillings are:

Sliced boiled egg with watercress
Low fat cheese and chutney
Tuna and tomatoes
Cottage cheese and pineapple
Chicken and gherkins
Turkey and cranberry sauce

Spicy Chicken Drumsticks

Ingredients:

4 chicken drumsticks, skinned
20g margarine
1 teaspoon mustard
½ tablespoon Worcestershire sauce
½ tablespoon tomato ketchup

Make several cuts on each chicken drumstick about 5mm long by 5mm deep. Cream the margarine with the mustard, Worcestershire sauce and ketchup. Spread the mixture over the drumsticks, then place them in a roasting tin. Roast in a preheated oven at 200°C (400°F, gas mark 6) for about 35 minutes, basting two or three times during cooking. Remove from the oven and allow to cool on some kitchen paper to drain off the fat.

Ginger Chicken Drumsticks

Ingredients:

4 chicken drumsticks, skinned
2 tablespoons soy sauce
1 tablespoon honey
½ teaspoon 5 spice powder
1 teaspoon grated fresh ginger
squeeze of lemon

Place the chicken drumsticks in a small baking dish. Mix together the remaining ingredients and pour over the drumsticks, coating well. Leave overnight to marinate. Cook in a preheated oven at 200°C (400°F, gas mark 6) for about 35 minutes, basting with the marinade from time to time. Remove from the oven and allow to cool. Drain off the fat on some kitchen paper.

French Tarragon Dressing

Ingredients:

2 tablespoons Dijon mustard
6 tablespoons olive oil
2 tablespoons tarragon vinegar
4 garlic cloves
1 tablespoon fresh parsley, chopped
2 tablespoons fresh tarragon, chopped
1 tablespoon anchovy essence
1 tablespoon tomato paste
¼ teaspoon sugar
salt and black pepper for seasoning

Peel and crush the cloves of garlic. Mix all the ingredients together. Store in an air tight bottle or jar in the refrigerator. Use as required.

Mackerel Salad

Ingredients:

135g penne
135g smoked mackerel fillets
1 medium size apple, diced
2 sticks of celery, chopped
squeeze of lemon juice
1 small bulb of fennel, diced
ground black pepper

Cook the penne in boiling water until tender. Flake the mackerel fillets into a small bowl, and squeeze a little lemon juice over the top. Season with the pepper. Add the penne and the remaining ingredients to the fish and mix together. Use a low calorie dressing when serving.

Avocado Salad

Ingredients:

Several lettuce leaves
1 small ripe avocado, peeled, stoned and diced
zest and juice of 1 lemon
175g bean-sprouts, washed
120g sweetcorn, cooked
50g button mushrooms, sliced

Place the diced avocado in a large bowl with the lemon juice and zest. Add the remaining ingredients and fold together. Serve on a bed of lettuce leaves.

Tuna and Penne Salad

Ingredients:

135g penne
1 x 200g tin tuna steaks, in brine
1 stick of celery, washed and thinly sliced
1 small head of broccoli, chopped small
25g seedless sultanas, washed
squeeze of lemon juice
mayonnaise, as required

Cook the penne in boiling water until tender. Flake the tuna steaks and place in a bowl. Add the rest of the ingredients and mix together. Gently fold the penne into the mixture. Squeeze a little lemon juice over the top, and if required a small amount of low-fat mayonnaise.

Egg and Tomato Salad

Ingredients:

a few lettuce leaves
3 salad tomatoes, sliced

3 or 4 spring onions, sliced
1 hard boiled egg, sliced
½ punnet of watercress
¼ cucumber, peeled and sliced
½ punnet mustard and cress
6 small radishes
1 tablespoon olive oil
1 tablespoon apple cider vinegar
seasoning for flavouring

Wash the vegetables, and break the lettuce leaves into small pieces and put into a salad bowl, with the cress, etc. Mix the oil and vinegar and flavour with salt, pepper. Sprinkle over the salad; garnish with sliced egg.

Spinach Salad

Ingredients:

250g fresh spinach, washed and shredded
10 water chestnuts, sliced
3 green onions, sliced
1 cup sliced mushrooms
1 cucumber, peeled and sliced
2 tablespoons olive oil
2 tablespoons soy sauce
3 tablespoons lemon juice
1½ tablespoons honey
1 tablespoon sesame seeds, toasted

Combine spinach, water chestnuts, green onions, mushrooms, and cucumber in a salad bowl. Mix together olive oil, soy sauce, lemon juice, and honey; pour over salad. Sprinkle with sesame seeds.

Apple and Pineapple Refresher

Ingredients:

1 litre apple juice
1½ cups unsweetened pineapple juice
2 tablespoons honey
2 tablespoons fresh lemon juice
3 cinnamon sticks

Mix all ingredients together in a saucepan. Heat until simmering over low heat. Remove the cinnamon sticks. Ladle the mixture into serving cups.

Potato Salad

Ingredients:

225g new potatoes, cooked and allowed to cool
1 teaspoon chopped parsley

1 tablespoon olive oil
1 tablespoon tarragon vinegar
a few capers
1 small onion, chopped
salt and pepper to season

Cut the potatoes into slices and put into a bowl with the chopped parsley, capers, and onion. Season with salt and pepper. Mix the oil and vinegar together, pour over the potatoes. Cooked butter beans or sliced beetroot is an alternative to onions and may be put in between the layers of potatoes.

Wild Mushroom Salad

Ingredients:

450g fresh wild mushrooms, sliced
1 teaspoon fresh tarragon
1 teaspoon fresh parsley
1 teaspoon fresh thyme
250g oakleaf and radicchio leaves
25g toasted pine nuts
3 salad tomatoes, peeled and diced
1 onion, chopped
5 tablespoons olive oil
50ml balsamic vinegar
salt and ground black pepper for seasoning

Peel and finely chop the onion. Season the balsamic vinegar with salt and pepper. Add four tablespoons of olive oil and whisk together in a mixing bowl. Pour into a jar or serving cruet and place to one side. Wash the lettuce and remove the leaves from the stalks. Pat the leaves dry. Heat the remaining olive oil in a large frying pan. Add the mushrooms to the pan and sauté until cooked. Add the herbs and vinaigrette to the mushrooms and stir together. Place the hot mushrooms in a bowl with the lettuce leaves and toss together. Add the pine nuts and diced tomatoes.

Avocado with Sweet Balsamic Vinaigrette

Ingredients:

1 lollo rosso lettuce
4 tomatoes
75ml balsamic vinegar
½ teaspoon celery salt
3 teaspoons granulated sugar
1 shallot
2 tablespoons olive oil
50g feta cheese
1 avocado

Wash and prepare the vegetables. Slice the tomatoes into quarters. Peel, stone and slice the avocado. Remove the lettuce leaves from the stalks, wash and pat dry. Peel and grate the shallot. Blend the balsamic vinegar with the celery salt, sugar, and grated shallot. Whisk all the ingredients together. Slowly add the olive oil while continuing to mix the dressing. Crumble the feta cheese over the salad before serving.

Celeriac and Pine Nut Salad

Ingredients:

1 lettuce
1 red onion, thinly sliced
3 tablespoons pine nuts
250g red cabbage, shredded
175g celeriac, shredded into matchstick lengths
50g seedless raisins
2 tablespoons balsamic vinegar
4 tablespoons olive oil

Wash and prepare the lettuce. Fry the red onion slices and pine nuts in two tablespoons of olive oil until the nuts are browned evenly and the onions are soft. Place the celeriac, red cabbage and raisins into a large bowl and mix in the onions and nuts. Pour the balsamic vinegar and remaining olive oil over the ingredients; toss the vegetables thoroughly to mix with the dressing. Place on a serving dish over a bed of crispy lettuce leaves.

Baked Beetroot Salad

Ingredients:

450g uncooked beetroots, peeled and quartered
1 red onion, peeled and chopped
2 cloves of garlic, peeled and crushed
100ml olive oil
1 tablespoon fresh oregano, chopped
1 tablespoon balsamic vinegar
1 tablespoon walnut oil
salt and pepper for seasoning

Combine the chopped red onion with the balsamic vinegar. Add the walnut oil and half of the olive oil to make a light dressing. Preheat the oven to 200°C (400°F, gas mark 6). Pour the rest of the olive oil into a roasting tin to cover the bottom. Add the beetroots and oregano. Season with salt and pepper. Roast the beetroots for forty-five minutes then add the garlic. Continue roasting for another forty minutes. Baste the beetroots with their own juices whilst cooking. Remove from the oven when the beetroots are tender. When cool chop the beetroots into small cubes or alternatively into slices. Place on a serving dish and pour the red onion dressing over the top.

Stuffed Capsicum

Ingredients:

4 red capsicum
1 onion, chopped
175g fennel, chopped
100g pine nuts
100g apricots, chopped
2 tablespoons mixed herbs
1 tablespoon balsamic vinegar
350g long grain rice
2 tablespoons olive oil
salt and ground black pepper for seasoning

Fry the onions and fennel in half the olive oil until soft. Stir in the pine nuts and continue frying until lightly golden brown. Add the apricots and herbs and cook for a further two minutes. Cook the rice in boiling water with the balsamic vinegar added to it. Drain well then mix the rice with the rest of the cooked ingredients. Season to taste. Core and de-seed the capsicum. Stuff with the rice mixture and replace the capsicum tops. Drizzle the rest of the olive oil over and place them in an oven dish. Bake in a preheated oven for twenty-five minutes at 180°C (350°F, gas mark 4). When ready place on a serving dish and serve immediately. Ideally serve whilst warm with a summer salad.

Vegetable Medley

Ingredients:

200g salad potatoes
100g carrots, sliced
2 small leeks, sliced
100g broccoli, sliced into florets
100g tomatoes
25ml balsamic vinegar

Wash and prepare the vegetables. Boil the carrots and potatoes in a large saucepan for five minutes. Add the broccoli and leeks, continue cooking until tender. Drain the vegetables, place in a serving dish and allow to cool. Cut the tomatoes into quarters and place on top of the vegetables. Drizzle the balsamic vinegar over the top before serving.

Artichokes in Balsamic Dressing

Ingredients:

1 lemon
3 artichokes

½ teaspoon salt
100g parmesan cheese, grated
red oak leaf lettuce leaves, prepared
1 tablespoon balsamic vinegar
50ml olive oil
salt and ground black pepper for seasoning

Prepare the artichokes first. Break off the stems removing the tough fibres from the centre of the base. Cut off the tough bottom leaves from the artichokes. Clip off the spiny tops of the other leaves. Carefully spread the leaves apart until you can see the inner central cone. Pull out the cone in one piece and scoop out the hairy fibres with a spoon.

Slice the lemon in half. With one half of the lemon, rub the juice into the sliced leaves to prevent them being discoloured. Squeeze the other half of the lemon into a bowl of cold water and plunge the artichokes into the water. Add the salt and some of the lemon juice to a pan of water (do not use an aluminium or iron pan). Gently boil the artichokes, uncovered for thirty to forty minutes. The leaves will easily pull off when cooked.

Place the lettuce leaves on a serving dish. Season with salt and pepper. Chop the artichokes and place on top of the lettuce. Sprinkle with parmesan cheese and drizzle the olive oil and balsamic vinegar over the top.

Chicken with California Pistachio Sauce

Ingredients:

4 chicken breasts
25g chopped pistachio nuts
2 spring onions
1 tablespoon olive oil
1 fresh orange
3 tablespoons water
3 teaspoons balsamic vinegar
salt and ground black pepper for seasoning

Squeeze the juice from the orange and keep to one side. Peel the onions and thinly slice crosswise. Wash the chicken breasts and pat them dry on a clean kitchen towel. Remove and discard the skin and bones.

Using a kitchen mallet or the flat side of a heavy knife, flatten the chicken breasts to 1cm (½ inch) thickness. Season with salt and black pepper. Place the chicken breasts in an oiled frying pan and fry on each side for two to three minutes until they are browned on both sides. Add the orange juice, water and balsamic vinegar to the pan, cover and simmer for ten minutes. Remove the chicken pieces to a serving dish and keep warm.

Place the spring onions and pistachio nuts in the same frying pan with the left-over juices, add a touch of olive oil and cook over medium heat until slightly thickened. Pour the sauce over the chicken and serve.

Honey Grilled Pork Chops

Ingredients:

4 boneless pork loin chops, about 25mm (1 inch) thick
150ml garlic vinegar
squeeze of lemon juice
1 tablespoon soy sauce
2 tablespoons honey
¼ teaspoon black pepper

Whisk together the garlic vinegar, soy sauce, honey and pepper. Add a squeeze of lemon juice. Flatten the pork chops with a meat mallet. Place in a shallow dish and pour the marinade over the chops. Cover the dish and marinate for four hours, turning the meat occasionally. Remove the pork chops from the marinade. Place under a hot grill and cook for ten to fifteen minutes, turning once and basting with the marinade.

Honey Glazed Onions

Ingredients:

450g small sweet onions
50g unsalted butter
3 tablespoons runny honey
squeeze of 1 lemon
salt and ground black pepper for seasoning
4 tablespoons fresh water

Peel the onions but leave whole. Melt the butter in a frying pan over a medium heat. Fry the onions for about five minutes or until the outside becomes brown in patches; be careful not to burn the butter. Season according to taste. Mix together the honey, water and lemon juice and pour over the onions. Allow to simmer until the onions are tender. If necessary add more water if required.

Grilled Chicken Slices

Ingredients:

4 boneless chicken breasts, about 25mm thick
25ml lemon juice
2 tablespoons honey
1 clove garlic, crushed
¼ teaspoon ground black pepper

Combine all the ingredients, except the chicken slices, to make a marinade. Mix well.

Place the chicken slices in a shallow dish and pour over the marinade. Cover and refrigerate for twenty-four hours, turning the chicken occasionally. Remove the chicken slices from the marinade. Place under a grill and cook for ten to fifteen minutes, turning once. Baste with the marinade whilst cooking.

Honey Baked Ham

Ingredients:

- 10 slices of honey baked ham
- 3 ripe nectarines
- 1 tablespoon fresh mint
- 1 teaspoon caster sugar
- 1 tablespoon mint vinegar
- 1 tablespoon raspberry vinegar
- 5 tablespoons olive oil
- salt and ground black pepper for seasoning

Place the mint and caster sugar in a mixing bowl and use a spoon to combine the mint with the caster sugar. Add the mint and raspberry vinegar and blend together. Add more sugar if necessary to sweeten. Stir in the olive oil. Slice the nectarines in half. Remove the pips and add to the dressing. Marinade the nectarines for one hour before serving. Arrange the nectarines on a serving dish and pour the marinade over. Serve with the honey baked ham.

Peach Glazed Pork Chops

Ingredients:

- 4 boneless pork loin chops, about 25mm thick
- 225ml peach vinegar
- 1 lemon
- 2 tablespoons soy sauce
- 2 tablespoons honey
- 1 clove of garlic, minced
- salt and pepper to taste

Flatten the loin chops with a meat mallet and place in a glass dish. Combine all the other ingredients and blend together. Pour the marinade over the chops and marinate for two hours. Remove pork chops from the marinade. Place under a preheated grill and grill for ten to fifteen minutes, turning once, baste with the marinade whilst cooking.

Chicken in Balsamic Sauce

Ingredients:

- 4 chicken breasts, skinned and boned
- 1 onion, chopped
- 1 tablespoon tomato paste
- 1 teaspoon sugar

5 tablespoons soy sauce
5 tablespoons balsamic vinegar
1 clove of garlic, crushed
olive oil
salt and ground black pepper for seasoning

Preheat the oven to 200°C (400°F, gas mark 6). Coat the chicken breasts and onion with olive oil, and season with salt and pepper. Combine the rest of the ingredients in a bowl and whisk thoroughly. Place the chicken breasts and chopped onion in a roasting pan and cook in the oven for thirty minutes. Pour the sauce over the chicken breasts and continue cooking for another twenty-five minutes basting frequently.

Spicy Chicken

Ingredients:

450g chicken thighs
1 teaspoon ginger, crushed
1 garlic clove, crushed
1 tablespoon sesame seed paste
1 tablespoon honey
½ teaspoon salt
2 tablespoons soy sauce
½ tablespoon red wine
1 tablespoon hot pepper oil
¼ teaspoon black pepper
coriander to taste
squeeze of lemon

Place the chicken and coriander to one side. Mix all the remaining ingredients in a saucepan and warm over a low heat. Stir to blend together. Place the chicken in a saucepan in enough water to cover. Boil over a high heat until thoroughly cooked. Prick the chicken with a fork to make sure it is cooked through and no pink juices flow out. Drain and allow to cool slightly. Bone the chicken and cut the meat into 5cm long by 1cm wide pieces. Arrange on a plate before serving. Pour the sauce over the chicken pieces, and garnish with coriander.

Chicken Livers on French Bread

Ingredients:

1 small onion, peeled and sliced
4 salad tomatoes, thickly sliced
100g chicken livers
1 tablespoon plain flour
1 French loaf
garlic butter, as required
2 tablespoons olive oil

1 teaspoon balsamic vinegar
2 tablespoons red wine
1 tablespoon fresh basil, chopped
salt and ground black pepper for seasoning

Prepare the chicken livers by rolling them in the plain flour. Heat the olive oil in a frying pan. Add the onion slices and sauté until golden brown. Add the chicken livers and fry over a medium heat until they are browned on all sides. Add the red wine and balsamic vinegar, bring to the boil, then simmer for a few minutes.

Remove from the pan to a mixing bowl and mash the chicken livers in the balsamic vinegar and red wine. Season with salt and pepper.

Slice the French loaf and spread with garlic butter. Warm under a grill or in a hot oven to melt the butter. Spread with chicken livers and tomatoes. Sprinkle some fresh chopped basil over the tomatoes.

Stir-fried Chicken in Balsamic Sauce

Ingredients:

4 chicken breasts, skinned and boned
1 stick celery, chopped
1 onion, sliced
2 garlic cloves, crushed
225g wild mushrooms
4 teaspoons soy sauce
4 teaspoons balsamic vinegar
2 teaspoons red wine
1 teaspoon sugar
2 tablespoons olive oil
salt and pepper according to taste

Mix the soy sauce, balsamic vinegar, sugar and red wine in a mixing bowl. Thinly slice the chicken breasts across the grain of the meat. Place the slices in the marinade and marinate for one hour. Clean and thinly slice the mushrooms. Heat the olive oil in large frying pan. Stir-fry the chicken slices until the juices run free and the meat changes colour. Add the vegetables, a little at a time, until all the ingredients are cooked. Add a little of the marinade while cooking. Serve with boiled rice and stir-fried vegetables.

Barbecued Fish

Ingredients:

4 fresh water fish

Marinade:

4 cloves garlic, crushed
1 tablespoon ginger, crushed
2 teaspoons sesame oil

3 tablespoons soy sauce
2 tablespoons sherry
1 tablespoon lemon juice, fresh
1 teaspoon honey

Remove the head and tail and gut the fish. Score the sides of the fish with deep cuts about 5cm (2 inches) apart on each side. Place the fish on a sheet of cooking foil.

Blend the marinade ingredients and poor over the fish. Cover and leave to marinate for 2 hours.

Barbecue the fish for 5 minutes or until well cooked on each side. Brush each fish with the marinade whilst it is cooking. May be served hot or cold on a serving dish.

Garlic Pork

Ingredients:

450g lean pork
2 tablespoons honey
2 teaspoons sesame oil

Sauce:

2 tablespoons sherry
4 tablespoons soy sauce
2 tablespoons Hoisin sauce
2 teaspoons honey
3 cloves garlic, crushed
2 teaspoons ginger, crushed

Slice the pork into 75mm (3 inch) x 25mm (1 inch) thin strips. Mix the sauce ingredients together and marinate the pork for at least 12 hours. Drain the pork from the marinade and place on a wire rack over a roasting tin half filled with water. Mix the sesame oil and honey and coat the pork pieces. Cook in a hot oven for 15 to 20 minutes. Turn over and baste on the other side and cook for a further 15 to 20 minutes.

Honey and Lemon Chicken Pieces

Ingredients:

450g chicken thighs, boned and skinned
1 lemon, thinly sliced
2 tablespoons honey
2 tablespoons sesame oil
2 tablespoons soy sauce
4 cloves garlic, crushed
1 tablespoon sesame seeds

Blend together all the ingredients except the chicken and sesame seeds. Add the chicken and mix well until the chicken is coated. Leave to marinate overnight. Place all the ingredients in an oven proof dish and cook for 40 minutes until the chicken is thoroughly cooked and is a golden brown colour. Baste the chicken during cooking. Serve on a dish garnished with green vegetables.

Barbecue Sauce

Ingredients:

3 tablespoons honey
2 tablespoons ketchup
50g butter
1 tablespoon vinegar
2 teaspoons Dijon style mustard
2 tablespoons brown sugar
1 tablespoon soy sauce
2 cloves garlic - crushed

Combine all the ingredients in a saucepan and simmer for 5 minutes. Makes about 1½ cups sauce. Leftovers can be stored in the refrigerator for later use.

Baked Beetroot Salad

Ingredients:

450g uncooked beetroots, peeled and quartered
1 red onion, peeled and chopped
2 cloves of garlic, peeled crushed
100ml olive oil
1 tablespoon fresh oregano, chopped
1 tablespoon balsamic vinegar
1 tablespoon walnut oil

Combine the chopped red onion with the balsamic vinegar. Add the walnut oil and half of the olive oil to make a light dressing. Preheat the oven to 200°C (400°F, gas mark 6). Pour the rest of the olive oil into a roasting tin to cover the bottom. Add the beetroots and oregano. Season with salt and pepper. Roast the beetroots for forty-five minutes then add the garlic. Continue roasting for another forty minutes. Baste the beetroots with their own juices whilst cooking. Remove from the oven when the beetroots are tender. When cool chop the beetroots into small cubes or alternatively into slices. Place on a serving dish and pour the red onion dressing over the top.

Beef Tomato Dressing

Ingredients:

2 beef tomatoes, chopped
4 spring onions, chopped
115g black olives, pitted and chopped
115g mild green chillies, chopped

3 tablespoons olive oil
1½ tablespoons white wine vinegar
garlic salt and ground black pepper for seasoning

Mix the beef tomatoes, spring onions, olives and chillies in a bowl. Blend in the olive oil, vinegar and seasoning to complete the dressing.

Aubergine Chutney

Ingredients:

3 aubergines
1 large onion
4 cloves fresh garlic
1 stick of celery
2 large pears
2 tablespoons olive oil
1 tablespoon tomato purée
1 tablespoon sugar
75ml white wine vinegar
75ml dry white wine
1 teaspoon capers
1 tablespoon sultanas
½ lemon
salt and ground black pepper for seasoning

Place the sultanas in a basin. Boil the white wine and pour over the sultanas. Cut the aubergines into small cubes and place in a colander. Sprinkle liberally with salt. Leave for about thirty minutes.

Finely chop the celery stick and onion and fry in a little olive oil until softened. Crush the garlic and add to the celery and onion. Season to taste then add the tomato purée. Peel and core the pears and cut the flesh into small cubes. Squeeze the lemon juice over the pears to stop discolouration. Coat the cubed pears with sugar in a basin. Empty the contents into a saucepan and cook over a low heat until the sugar begins to caramelise. Add the white wine vinegar and continue cooking until dry. Fry the aubergines in the remaining olive oil until golden brown. Add the cooked vegetables and fruit and mix in the white wine and sultanas. Cover the pan and cook very gently for thirty minutes or until the mixture has thickened. Add the capers and season to taste. Store in a jar with an air tight lid and keep refrigerated. This is a delicious chutney especially when served with pitta bread or toast.

Grilled Mullet in White Wine

Ingredients:

3 red mullet, cleaned
3 teaspoons toasted fennel seeds, crushed

lemon juice
2 tablespoons olive oil
6 cloves of garlic, sliced
1 beef tomato, thinly sliced
4 tablespoons groundnut oil
2 tablespoons white wine
salt and ground black pepper for seasoning

Slice the fish lightly on each side and stuff the slits with the crushed fennel seeds. Coat the fish with olive oil and squeeze the lemon juice over the top. Place in a grill pan with the slices of garlic between the fish. Grill under a high heat for five minutes then reduce the heat and continue cooking for a further four to five minutes on each side. Baste with some more of the olive oil whilst cooking. When cooked, bone the fish. Serve on individual plates with the sliced tomatoes. Sprinkled the garlic over the top of the fish. Season with salt and pepper. Mix the groundnut oil with the white wine until thoroughly blended. Pour over the fish before serving.

Chicken Breasts in Lime Juice

Ingredients:

4 chicken breasts, skinned and boned
2 tablespoons plain flour
1 tablespoon olive oil
75g unsalted butter
1 tablespoon chervil
1 tablespoon dill
1 tablespoon parsley
1 tablespoon chives
1 tablespoon basil
1 tablespoon mint
1 tablespoon rosemary
3 cloves garlic
¼ teaspoon chilli paste
1 lime
4 tablespoons chicken stock
4 tablespoons white wine
salt and ground black pepper for seasoning

Grate the rind of the lime and squeeze out the juice. Peel and finely chop the cloves of garlic. Roll the chicken breasts in the plain flour. Heat the olive oil in a large frying pan. Place the chicken breasts in the oil and fry over a medium heat turning to seal the meat on all sides. Remove from the pan and keep warm. Place the butter, chilli paste and all the herbs in the frying pan together with the lime juice, grated rind, chicken stock and white wine. Bring the liquid to a boil then add the chicken breasts. Cover the frying pan and continue cooking for a further ten minutes or until the chicken is cooked right through. Season with salt and pepper. Pour the sauce over the chicken breasts before serving.

Tagliatelle, Garlic and Mushrooms

Ingredients:

350g chicken breast, cooked and diced
25g butter
1 onion, sliced
1 tablespoon olive oil
3 cloves of garlic, crushed
175g button mushroom
3 tablespoons dry sherry
2 teaspoons white wine
200ml creme fraiche
salt and pepper for seasoning
1 tablespoon parsley, chopped
350g tagliatelle

Heat the butter and oil in a frying pan. Sauté the onion and garlic until soft. Add the chicken to the pan and fry for a further five minutes. In the meantime, cook the tagliatelle in boiling salted water for ten to twelve minutes. Add the mushrooms to the chicken and fry for five minutes. Stir in the sherry, white wine, creme fraiche and seasoning. Cook gently for two to three minutes. Drain the pasta and serve topped with the chicken and sauce. Sprinkle liberally with the chopped parsley.

Fagioli Bean Casserole

Ingredients:

100g fagioli beans
3 fresh garlic clove, crushed
1 onion, sliced
200g tinned plum tomatoes, chopped
150g fresh tomatoes
200ml fresh apple juice
2 tablespoons white wine
1 teaspoon syrup
1 teaspoon demerara sugar
salt and ground black pepper for seasoning

Soak the beans overnight or for at least eight hours. Drain and rinse thoroughly. Place in a large saucepan, cover and boil for ten minutes, reduce the heat and cook for a further five minutes. Drain the beans and rinse. Place the fresh tomatoes in boiling water for ten minutes, remove and sieve to remove the seeds and skins. Mix together the apple juice, white wine, syrup and demerara sugar. Place all ingredients into a large casserole dish and cook on medium for forty minutes. Stirring occasionally. Add some water if necessary to prevent the beans from becoming too dry. Season to taste.

Lemon Pepper Dressing

Ingredients:

50ml white wine
1 tablespoon vegetable oil
3 cloves of garlic
2 teaspoons honey
1 unwaxed lemon
salt and ground black pepper for seasoning

Peel the cloves of garlic and put the cloves through a mincer. Grate the lemon peel, being careful not to include any of the pith. Squeeze the lemon and put 50ml of the juice to one side. Combine all the ingredients, mixing well. This is an excellent dressing for cooked French beans: remember to drizzle over whilst the beans are still warm. It is also an ideal dressing for salads.

Grilled Lamb Chops

Ingredients:

8 small lamb chops
4 garlic cloves
1 red capsicum, chopped
1 yellow capsicum, chopped
175g courgettes
75ml olive oil
45ml red wine
½ teaspoon sugar
salt and ground black pepper for seasoning

Wash and prepare the vegetables. Chop the capsicum into 1cm squares. Slice the courgettes and cloves of garlic. Whisk together the sugar, olive oil, and red wine. Preheat the grill. Place the chops and the vegetables under the grill and cook for ten minutes or until the meat and vegetables have browned. Turn the vegetables and chops over and continue cooking on the other side until the meat is tender. Whilst cooking, drizzle the sauce over the vegetables and meat. Season with salt and pepper.

French Bread Salad

Ingredients:

3 slices French bread
175g Italian marinated dried tomatoes
350g tomatoes
½ cucumber

1 red onion
2 tablespoons red wine
1 tablespoon water
3 cloves garlic
1 teaspoon dried mixed herbs
salt and ground black pepper for seasoning

Preheat the oven to 180°C (350°F, gas mark 4). Cut the French bread slices into 25mm cubes and place on a baking sheet in a single layer. Bake for ten minutes or until lightly browned; turn over whilst baking to brown all sides. Remove from the oven and set aside. Drain the oil from the marinated tomatoes into a small bowl. Wash and pat dry the fresh vegetables. Cut the tomatoes into quarters. Peel the cucumber and dice into large chunks. Peel the onion and garlic and finely chop into small pieces. Place all the vegetables and herbs into a large bowl. Add the red wine and water and stir well to combine. Season with salt and pepper. Before serving pour the tomato oil over and toss the vegetables. Sprinkle the bread cubes over or alternatively toss with the rest of the salad.

Salsa

Ingredients:

1 red onion
1 green capsicum
2 cloves garlic
1 tablespoon olive oil
450g fresh tomatoes
½ teaspoon fresh oregano
35ml red wine
2 tablespoons fresh thyme
salt and ground black pepper for seasoning

Wash and prepare the vegetables. Chop the onion, tomatoes and capsicum. Chop the thyme and oregano very finely or use dried prepared herbs. Crush the cloves of garlic.

Heat the olive oil in a large pan. Fry the red onion until soft then add the rest of the vegetables except the tomatoes and herbs. Cook until all the vegetables are soft. Add the tomatoes, red wine and herbs and continue cooking for another five minutes. Season with salt and pepper. Leave in a refrigerator overnight to blend all the flavours together. A versatile sauce to use in recipes with eggs, roast pork, fish and salads. Store in a refrigerator for up to seven days.

Fried Halibut In Red Wine

Ingredients:

225g halibut fillets, 2cm thick

100g plain white flour
150ml olive oil
3 tomatoes, peeled and chopped
100ml red wine
4 cloves fresh garlic, minced
1 tablespoon dried rosemary, crumbled
2 teaspoons dried thyme, crumbled
3 bay leaves
salt and ground black pepper for seasoning

Wash the halibut fillets in cold water and pat dry. Sprinkle with salt and pepper and coat with plain flour. Heat half the olive oil in a shallow pan. Add the fish a little at a time and fry for two minutes each side. Drain on paper towels. Add the remaining olive oil to the same pan and add all the remaining ingredients. Simmer over a low heat stirring frequently for about fifteen minutes until the liquid has evaporated and the sauce has thickened. Arrange the fish on a serving dish and pour the sauce over.

Duck Breasts in Orange Sauce

Ingredients:

4 duck breasts
3 tablespoons olive oil
4 tablespoons red wine
1 tablespoon soy sauce
2 tablespoons morello cherry conserve
4 cloves of garlic, crushed
1 orange
1 teaspoon cornflour
3 tablespoons chicken stock
salt and ground black pepper for seasoning

Peel and crush the cloves of garlic. Place the olive oil in a small saucepan with the soy sauce, red wine and morello jelly conserve. Gently heat the sauce stirring all the time until smooth. Wash the duck breasts. Remove the skin and bones. Place in a refrigerator container and marinate in the sauce for one hour. Prepare four squares of cooking foil large enough to wrap each piece of duck breast. Place one breast in each piece of foil. Squeeze the orange juice and a little of the sauce over the duck, season well, and fold the foil into parcels. Heat the oven to 200°C (400°F, gas mark 6). Place the wrapped duck parcels on a baking tin or tray and cook on the top rack in the oven for 25 minutes. Whisk the chicken stock with the cornflour. Reheat the marinade, add the chicken stock and simmer until reduced down by half. Before serving unwrap the duck breasts and place on a serving dish. Drizzle the sauce over the duck.

Spinach Quiche

Ingredients:

250g wholemeal shortcrust pastry
30ml olive oil
1 large onion, sliced
2 courgettes, diced
1 large carrot, diced
75g button mushrooms, quartered
100g spinach, cooked, drained and chopped
pinch of nutmeg
100g cashew nuts, chopped
1 large tomato, cut into thin wedges
3 eggs
60ml skimmed milk
½ teaspoon mixed herbs
100g Cheddar cheese
50g grated mozzarella cheese
salt and pepper

Roll out the pastry and line into a 23cm flan tin. Chill for 30 minutes. Set the oven to 200°C (400°F, gas mark 6) and bake the pastry case blind for 20 minutes. Heat the oil in a frying pan and sauté the onion slices until soft. Add the courgettes, carrot and mushrooms and cook until just softened. Season the spinach with nutmeg, salt and pepper, and spread into the pastry case; then spoon over the cooked vegetables. Scatter over the cashew nuts and arrange the tomato wedges on top. Whisk together the eggs, milk and herbs. Pour into the flan case, sprinkle with the cheeses and bake for 20 minutes. Reduce the oven temperature to 180°C (350°F, gas mark 4) and bake for a further 15 to 20 minutes or until set.

Spaghetti à l'Italienne

Ingredients:

For the sauce:
4 tomatoes, chopped
250ml water
salt and cayenne pepper for seasoning
15g flour
1 small onion, chopped finely
25g minced ham
squeeze of lemon juice

Put the onion, tomatoes, and ham into a saucepan, with the water. Allow to simmer until tender. Add the flour blended with a little water. Add the lemon juice, cayenne pepper, and salt. Cook for two minutes, stirring well.

Main ingredients:

150g spaghetti
25g margarine
50g Cheddar cheese, grated
1 teaspoon grated parmesan cheese
salt and pepper for seasoning

Cook the spaghetti in boiling salted water, then strain. Add the margarine and shake well over a low heat. Stir in the sauce, seasonings and grated cheeses. Serve on a hot dish.

Baked Vegetable Rice

Ingredients:

30g margarine
1 onion, chopped
½ teaspoon curry powder
100g brown rice
25g blanched almonds, slivered
30g red lentils
30g currants, washed
30g dried apricots, chopped
275ml chicken or vegetable stock
3 tablespoons fromage frais

Preheat the oven to 190°C (375°F, gas mark 5). Melt the margarine in a pan and gently sauté the onion until soft. Add the curry powder, rice and almonds and stir for one minute. Turn the rice mixture into a heatproof dish. Stir in the lentils and dried fruit, and pour on the stock. Cover the dish and bake for 40 minutes. Lightly fork the fromage frais into the rice and vegetables, and serve whilst still hot.

Cauliflower Soup

Ingredients:

1 medium size cauliflower, washed
2 medium size onions, finely chopped
600ml chicken stock
1 bay leaf
sprig of parsley
salt and pepper
pinch of grated nutmeg
300ml low-fat bio yoghurt
paprika for garnishing

Put the onion, stock and cauliflower into a pan. Add the bay leaf, parsley, salt and pepper, cover the pan, and cook for 10 to 15 minutes until the cauliflower is tender. Remove the bay leaf and purée the soup in a blender. Return to the pan, add the nutmeg and half of the yoghurt. Reheat without boiling. Serve with the remaining yoghurt and paprika.

Tomato Soup
Ingredients:

1 x 400g tin of tomatoes
1 onion
250ml milk
1 rasher of lean bacon
600ml vegetable stock
1 tablespoon flour
1 bay leaf
sprig of parsley, chopped
pepper and salt for seasoning

Place the bacon, cut into small pieces, in a pan, and add the onion. Place the lid on the pan and fry, shaking constantly for 1 minute. Add the tomatoes, bay leaf, parsley and stock. Bring to the boil, and then simmer for 30 minutes. Remove the bay leaf and purée the soup in a blender. Return to the pan. Mix the flour with the milk, add to the soup and stir till boiling. Add pepper and salt to season.

Onion and Lentil Soup
Serves 2-4

2 onions, chopped
1 tablespoon vegetable oil
1 medium sized carrot, chopped small
600ml vegetable stock
225g lentils, soaked overnight and drained
yeast extract
salt and pepper

Sauté the onions in the oil, add the carrot, lentils and vegetable stock, and cook until soft. Add the seasoning and yeast extract according to taste.

Leek and Lentil Soup
Serves 2-4

200g leeks
3 teaspoons of vegetable oil
½ litre vegetable stock
100g red lentils
salt for seasoning
bouquet garni

Sauté the leeks in the oil in a covered pan for ten minutes, stirring frequently. Add the stock, lentils, salt and a bouquet garni. Simmer for 30 minutes. When the lentils are soft, remove the bouquet garni. Serve whilst still hot.

Tagliatelle with Vegetables and Ham

Serves 2

1 teaspoon olive oil
2 cloves of garlic, crushed
1 small onion, chopped
1 courgette, chopped
½ red pepper, diced
50g button mushrooms, wiped and sliced
25g ham, chopped
100g tinned tomatoes, drained and mashed
salt and pepper for seasoning
200g tagliatelle
boiling water, salted
chopped parsley
Parmesan cheese

Cook the onions and garlic in the oil for 1 minute. Add the courgette, red pepper, and mushrooms; cover with a tight lid and cook for 2 minutes. Add the ham and tomatoes, cover and cook for 1½ minutes. Season to taste. Put to one side and keep warm.

Place the tagliatelle in a deep pot, and just cover with boiling, salted water. Add a few drops of oil to the water. Cover and cook for 4 minutes. Let the pot stand covered, while you reheat the sauce if necessary. Drain the tagliatelle, pour on the sauce, sprinkle with parsley and serve with Parmesan cheese.

Rice Risotto

Serves 2

1 tablespoon olive oil
1 onion, skinned and finely chopped
½ green pepper, finely diced
1 tablespoon tomato purée
2 cloves of garlic, crushed
salt and pepper for seasoning
180g brown rice
1 tablespoon wild rice
450ml hot chicken stock
50g boned cooked chicken, chopped
25g cooked ham, chopped
chopped fresh parsley, for garnishing

Place the olive oil, onion, pepper, tomato purée, garlic, and seasoning in a large covered microwave bowl. Cover and cook for 1 minute on high. Stir half way through cooking. Stir in the rice, hot chicken stock, chicken and ham. Re-cover the bowl and cook for a further 12 to 14 minutes. Leave to stand covered for 3 minutes, before serving. Garnish with chopped parsley.

Macaroni with Tuna

Serves 2

For the sauce:

25g margarine
3 tablespoons flour
150ml milk
20g Parmesan cheese
salt and pepper for seasoning

Put the margarine in a bowl and cook for 30 seconds. Stir in the flour and cook for 30 seconds. Stir in the milk and cook for 2 minutes, whisking after each minute. Stir in the cheese and cook for 30 seconds. Whisk again and season to taste. Keep warm.

Main ingredients:

200g macaroni
boiling water
olive oil
100g tinned tuna, in brine, drained and flaked
slices of red and green peppers to garnish

Put the macaroni in a deep pot and just cover with boiling water. Add a pinch of salt and a few drops of oil. Cover and cook for 7 minutes. Let the pot stand, covered, for 3 minutes. Drain the macaroni, stir in the sauce and tuna fish and heat through for 1-2 minutes. Garnish with the pepper slices and serve hot.

Turkey Cutlets

Serves 2

225g cooked turkey, light and dark meat
1 medium size onion, chopped
1 clove of garlic, crushed
1 tablespoon olive oil
1 teaspoon cornflour
75ml chicken stock
25g fresh breadcrumbs
½ teaspoon chopped fresh thyme
1 tablespoon low fat yoghurt
salt and pepper for seasoning

For coating:

1 egg white, lightly beaten
25g crisp breadcrumbs
2 tablespoons olive oil, for frying

Mince all the turkey meat. Sauté the onions and garlic in the olive oil until soft, stir in the cornflour and blend well. Add the stock, then bring to the boil. Stir over a moderate heat until a thick sauce is formed. Add the fresh breadcrumbs, thyme, yoghurt, turkey meat, and seasoning. Allow the mixture to become quite cold and firm. Form into 4 cutlet shapes. Brush with the egg white and coat in crisp breadcrumbs. Heat the oil and fry the cutlets on both sides until golden brown. Drain on kitchen paper.

Sweet & Sour Cabbage Cannelloni

Serves 2

- 150g green cabbage, shredded
- 20g unsalted butter
- 1 small onion, chopped
- 1 clove of garlic, crushed
- 1 small carrot, grated
- 1 apple, peeled, cored and grated
- salt, as required
- 300g ripe tomatoes, skinned and quartered
- 1 teaspoon brown sugar
- 2 teaspoons white wine vinegar
- 20g raisins
- 4 cannelloni tubes
- 75ml unsalted chicken stock

Prepare the cabbage stuffing: sauté the onion and garlic in the butter. Stir in the cabbage, carrot, apple, and a little salt to season. Add enough water to the pan so it is 5mm deep. Cover and steam for about 30 minutes. Set the pan aside. Pour 3 tablespoons of water into a saucepan over a medium heat. Add the tomatoes and cook, stirring often until soft, and the liquid has reduced - about 20 minutes. Purée the tomatoes in a bowl. Stir in the brown sugar, vinegar, raisins, season with salt.

Prepare the cannelloni: add the tubes to 1 litre of salted boiling water. Test after 15 minutes and cook until they are soft. Use a slotted spoon to transfer to a large bowl of cold water. Preheat the oven to 200°C (400°F, gas mark 6). Drain the cannelloni and fill each one equally with the cabbage stuffing. Arrange the tubes on a single layer in a large baking dish. Pour the stock over and cover tightly with foil. Bake for 30 minutes. Ten minutes before serving transfer the sauce from the bowl to a saucepan, and then bring to the boil. Reduce heat and simmer while the cannelloni finishes cooking. Serve the cannelloni immediately, with the sauce separately.

Tagliatelle with Mushroom Provençale

Serves 2

- 2 teaspoons olive oil
- 1 medium onion, chopped
- 2 cloves of garlic, crushed
- ½ teaspoon mixed fresh thyme and sage, chopped

2 large, ripe tomatoes, peeled and halved, seeded and finely chopped
225g button mushrooms
125g tagliatelle, cooked and drained

Sauté the onion and garlic in the oil for 2 minutes. Stir in the herbs, tomatoes, and mushrooms. Cook for a further 3 to 4 minutes. Serve the tagliatelle whilst hot, with the sauce poured over the top.

Beef Paprika

Serves 2

2 x 150g boneless sirloin steaks, trimmed of fat and cut in half
1 tablespoon paprika
1 tablespoon flour
2 tablespoons olive oil
1 small onion, roughly chopped
½ green pepper, sliced into 2cm squares
2 cloves of garlic, finely chopped
150ml chicken stock
50g flat mushrooms, cut into quarters
salt and pepper for seasoning

Season the pieces of beef with the salt and pepper. Combine half of the paprika and all the flour on a plate. Dredge the pieces of beef in this mixture, ensuring that each one is evenly coated. Reserve the remaining flour-paprika mixture. Seal the steaks in 1 tablespoon of hot oil in a non-stick pan. Wipe the pan clean with a paper towel; heat the remaining tablespoon of oil, and sauté the onion, green pepper and garlic for about 5 minutes, or until the onions are translucent. Add the remaining flour-paprika mixture, then whisk in the stock.

Add the meat and bring the stock to simmer. Cover the pan and simmer the beef and vegetables for 1¼ hours. Stir in the mushrooms and the remaining half of the paprika; cook the mixture, covered, for 15 minutes longer. Serve the beef surrounded by the vegetables and covered with the sauce.

Lamb Curry

Serves 2

2 teaspoons olive oil
1 onion, chopped
2 cloves of garlic, crushed
1 bay leaf
1 dessert spoonful curry powder
1 teaspoon ground turmeric
125g boneless lean lamb, cut into cubes
2 tomatoes, skinned and puréed
60g sultanas

2 teaspoons red wine vinegar
salt for seasoning
1 teaspoon garam masala
100g cauliflower florets, cut into small pieces
100g French beans, cut in half
100g long grain rice
50ml low fat yoghurt
water for cooking

Heat the oil over a medium heat in a heavy saucepan. Sauté the onion and garlic, bay leaf and half of the curry powder and turmeric, stirring occasionally, for about 5 minutes. Stir in the lamb and cook for 2 to 3 minutes, or until browned on all sides. Stir in 225ml of water, the tomato purée, sultanas, vinegar, and remaining curry powder and turmeric. Bring to the boil, cover and simmer for 45 minutes, or until the lamb is tender. Stir in the garam masala during the last five minutes of cooking.

While the lamb is cooking, bring 25mm of water to the boil in a medium-sized saucepan. Place the cauliflower and beans in a vegetable steamer and steam until just tender; remove from the pan and set aside. Bring 300ml of water to the boil in a saucepan, stir in the rice, cover, reduce the heat to low, and cook for 20 minutes, or until the water is absorbed. Place in a serving dish and keep warm.

When the lamb is tender, add the cauliflower and beans, cover and simmer for a further 5 minutes, or until heated through. Remove the pan from the heat; remove and discard the bay leaf. Stir the yoghurt into the curry and add seasoning.

Glazed Ham

Serves 6

Ingredients:

1.5 kg piece of ham, boned and rolled
1 bay leaf
a few peppercorns and cloves
3 tablespoons clear honey
juice of one orange
1 tablespoon cornflour
Pinch of salt and pepper

Place the ham in a large saucepan and add the bay leaf, peppercorns and cloves. Add water to cover and bring to the boil. Reduce the heat and simmer for about an hour. Drain and retain the liquid for stock. Place the ham in a roasting tin and score the rind into a diamond pattern. Mix the honey and fruit juice and pour over the joint allowing it to soak into the incisions. Season with salt and pepper. Roast in the Oven at 350° F/gas Mark 4 for about an hour or until tender. Remove the joint from the pan and serve with gravy made from stock blended with cornflour and allowed to boil until thick.

Ginger Sponge with Pineapple

Serves 2

200g pineapple chunks
75g butter
75g demerara sugar
1 egg
50g self raising flour
3 tablespoons of milk
½ teaspoon baking powder
1 teaspoon ground ginger

Place half the butter with half of the sugar in a heatproof bowl and cook on high for 45 seconds to caramelise, then arrange two thirds of the pineapple in the bottom of the bowl.

Beat the rest of the butter and sugar together, beat in the egg, fold in the flour, ginger and baking powder, then add the milk and the remaining pineapple. Spoon the mixture into the bowl with the pineapple and caramel. Cook for 4 minutes on high. Allow to stand for 8 minutes before serving.

Banana Cake

450g plain strong flour
1 teaspoon baking soda
1 teaspoon salt
100g unsalted butter
250g sugar
2 eggs
1 ripe banana, mashed
1 tablespoon milk
1 tablespoon white wine vinegar

Sift together the flour, salt and baking soda. Cream the butter and sugar, add the eggs one at a time and beat until fluffy. Add flour mixture alternately with bananas, milk and white wine vinegar. Whisk after each addition. Bake at 180°C (350°F, gas mark 4) for 60 minutes or until the top is brown and crispy.

Ginger Bread

450g plain strong flour
250g sugar
100g unsalted butter
1 egg
½ teaspoon ginger
1 teaspoon cinnamon

2 tablespoons molasses
1 teaspoon baking soda
275ml milk
1 tablespoon white wine vinegar
pinch of salt

Add the white wine vinegar to the milk to sour it. Mix together the flour, sugar, cinnamon and ginger. Mix in the butter and kneed with the fingers until the mixture is crumbly. Remove half and set to one side. Add to half the mixture, the molasses, egg, baking soda, pinch of salt and soured milk. Stir well. Pour ingredients into a greased 20cm x 20cm square pan. Sprinkle the top with the remaining mixture. Bake in an oven at 180°C (350°F, gas mark 4) for forty-five minutes.

Raisin Muffins

2 eggs
570ml fresh milk
100ml olive oil
4 tablespoons white wine vinegar
200g bran flour
100g raisins
1kg plain flour
350g sugar
1 teaspoon salt
1½ teaspoons baking soda

Whisk the milk, oil, white wine vinegar, and eggs in a large mixing bowl. Add the rest of ingredients and stir until blended. Bake in a preheated oven 180°C (350°F, gas mark 4) for twenty-five minutes. Raisin muffins can be stored in a refrigerator for up to ten days. Delicious eaten when still warm spread with butter and honey.

Ginger Bread Slices

450g plain flour
1 teaspoon baking soda
½ teaspoon salt
1½ teaspoons ginger
½ teaspoon ground cloves
½ teaspoon allspice
¼ teaspoon cinnamon
¼ teaspoon mace
100g unsalted butter
100g demerara sugar
100ml golden syrup
2 eggs
2 tablespoons white wine vinegar
100ml fresh milk

Sift the dry ingredients together in a mixing bowl. Place the syrup, sugar and butter into a saucepan and warm gently until melted. Mix into the dry ingredients. In a separate basin, beat together the milk, eggs and vinegar and add gradually to the mixture, mixing thoroughly. Place the mixture into a greased and floured 22cm x 33cm baking tin. Preheat the oven to 180°C (350°F, gas mark 4) and bake for twenty-five minutes or until well browned. Cut into 5cm x 10cm slices when cool.

Iced Gingerbread Biscuits

Ingredients:

1 cup butter
¾ cup brown sugar
¼ cup light corn syrup
¾ cup honey
1 teaspoon grated lemon rind
1 teaspoon vanilla extract
1 teaspoon ground ginger
½ teaspoon ground cloves
1 teaspoon ground cinnamon
1 teaspoon salt
1 teaspoon baking soda
4 to 4½ cups flour, sifted

Decorating Icing:

1½ cups sifted icing sugar
1 egg white
1 teaspoon lemon juice
few drops vanilla extract
food colourings

Cream the butter and sugar. Add syrup, honey, lemon rind and vanilla, spices, salt and soda. Add enough flour to make a soft dough. Chill until firm enough to roll out. Set the oven at 180°C (350°F, gas mark 4). Grease and flour baking sheets. Roll dough. Cut into desired shapes with pastry cutters. Bake for 8 minutes or until puffed and dry. Blend the sugar, egg white, lemon juice and vanilla together until the mixture stands in peaks. If necessary, add a little more sugar or egg white. Cover the bowl with a damp cloth when not being used. Divide the icing into separate bowls and add a different colour to each bowl. Stir until the colour is well mixed. Ice the biscuits.

Banana Bake

Ingredients:

4 large bananas
50g butter
2 tablespoons honey
lemon juice
sour cream

Peel the bananas and cut them in half lengthways. Set the oven to 180°C (350°F, gas mark 4). Grease a baking dish. Arrange banana halves in the dish. Dot with the butter, spread the honey and lemon juice over the bananas. Bake for 15 minutes. Put the sour cream into a bowl and serve it with your baked bananas.

Party Biscuits

Ingredients:

¼ cup shortening
¼ cup sugar
1 egg
¾ cup honey
1 teaspoon lemon flavouring
2¾ cups flour
1 teaspoon baking soda
1 teaspoon salt

Mix shortening, sugar, egg, honey and flavouring. Blend in the flour, soda and salt. Chill the dough. Roll the dough out and cut into shapes. Place 1 inch apart on greased flat sheet. Bake at 190°C (375°F, gas mark 5) until done.

Glazed Carrots

Ingredients:

1 bunch carrots
¼ cup melted butter or oleo
1 ½ teaspoon grated orange peel and lemon peel
Pinch of salt
¼ cup honey

Wash and scrape carrots. Cook in 1 inch boiling water for about 15 to 20 minutes until tender-crisp. Then drain. Blend the salt, melted butter, honey and grated peels. Pour mixture over the cooked carrots. Warm over a low heat until the carrots are thoroughly glazed.

Forrester's Jam

Ingredients:

1 cup berries
¼ cup honey
1 tablespoon lemon juice

Mash the berries in a pan and heat to a boil. Add the honey and lemon juice. Bring to a good rolling boil and cook at this temperature for 5 to 10 minutes or until it begins to thicken. This jam can be made over the camp stove, even while on a back-packing trip.

Easter Bread

Ingredients:

400g packet bread roll mix
½ cup golden raisins
1 teaspoon grated lemon peel
1 cup hot water (110 to 120 degrees)
2 tablespoons butter, softened
¼ teaspoon almond extract
1 large egg

Topping:

¼ cup honey
¼ cup butter, softened
2 tablespoons sliced almonds
coloured hard boiled eggs if desired

Using a large mixing bowl, combine the yeast with the flour mixture; mix well. Add raisins, lemon peel, water, 2 tablespoons butter, almond extract and egg; stir until dough pulls clean away from sides of bowl. Turn dough onto lightly floured surface.

With greased hands shape dough into ball. Knead dough for 5 minutes until smooth. Cover dough In large bowl and let rest 5 minutes. Grease large flat tin. Divide dough in 3 parts. On lightly floured surface, shape each into a 60cm rope. Braid ropes loosely from centre to each end. Place on cookie sheet and shape into a circle; pinch ends together to seal.

Heat the oven to 190°C (375°F, gas mark 5). Let dough rise on top of oven for about 30 minutes, then bake for 14-18 minutes or until the rolls are light brown.

Combine honey and ¼ cup butter and brush 2 tablespoons over braid after removing from oven. Arrange almonds on braid. Return to oven for 5 minutes. Remove from oven and cool on wire rack. Serve remaining mixture as an accompaniment to bread. Garnish centre of bread with coloured eggs.

Nut Candy

Ingredients:

400g dark honey
400g shelled walnuts, coarsely chopped
½ teaspoon ground ginger, or to taste
1 tablespoon lemon juice
1 tablespoon grated orange rind, optional
Vegetable oil, for platter

Place honey in heavy saucepan; bring to simmer over a low heat. Stir frequently with wooden spoon. Add nuts, ginger, lemon juice; orange rind if desired. Continue to simmer for ½ hour, or until honey reaches a dark brown colour, and walnuts have absorbed honey. Turn out the mixture onto a greased platter and spread evenly. Let stand until cool.

Coffee Cake

Ingredients:

- 1 cup cold black coffee
- 3 eggs
- 1 cup sugar
- 3 tablespoons oil
- 400g honey
- 3 cups flour
- 2 teaspoons baking powder
- 1 teaspoon baking soda
- ½ teaspoon cinnamon
- 1 teaspoon lemon juice
- 3 tablespoons orange marmalade

Beat with mixer oil, sugar, and eggs. Mix coffee and honey together. Sift dry ingredients together and add alternately with coffee and honey to the oil and sugar mixture. Add marmalade and lemon juice. Bake for about 45 minutes at 180°C (350°F, gas mark 4).

Honey Surprise

Ingredients:

- 100g raisins
- 25g dates
- 10g orange peel
- 10g lemon peel
- 50g dried figs
- 50g almond flour
- 15 ml orange juice
- 60 ml brandy
- 30 ml dark rum
- cinnamon cloves, to taste
- Star anise
- 50g rye flour
- 75ml milk
- 5g fresh yeast

One week prior to use, chop ingredients to the size of currants. Combine all ingredients except the flour, milk and yeast in an airtight container and store in a cool place. Mix flour, milk and yeast to make a dough and let it rise. Form the mixture into desired shape (no higher than 2cm). Garnish with whole almonds and bake at 170°C (325°F, gas mark 3) for approximately ½ hour. When cooked, brush with a syrup made of espresso and honey, and garnish with dried candied fruit. Wrap up when cool and store in an airtight box.

Pumpkin Pudding With Pecan Sauce

Ingredients:

¾ cup honey
2 teaspoons pumpkin pie spice
1½ cup canned pumpkin
1 cup evaporated skimmed milk
6 egg whites

Preheat oven to 180°C (350°F, gas mark 4). Combine honey, pumpkin, spice and milk in a mixing bowl; blend well. Beat the egg whites to stiff peaks; fold into pumpkin mixture. Pour into 6 soufflé dishes. Place in large baking dish that is filled with hot water almost to the top of the soufflé dishes. Bake 45-50 minutes or until knife inserted in the centre comes out clean. Remove warm pudding onto dessert plates; top with honey sauce. Garnish with lemon curls and mint leaves if desired. Mix ¼ cup honey and ½ cup pecan halves; stir in ¼ - ½ teaspoon rum flavouring. Spoon over warm pudding.

Yuletide Punch

Ingredients:

2 cartons orange juice
1 carton pineapple juice
½ cup honey
1 bottle soda water or lemonade
¼ cup lemon juice
vodka
sherbet ice cream (lime & cherry)
cherries

Combine orange juice, pineapple juice, honey, lemon juice and vodka. Drop ice cream scoops into punch bowl and cherries. Pour soda water or lemonade on top of ice cream so that it fizzes.

Honey Biscuits

Ingredients:

¼ cup soft shortening
¼ cup white sugar
1 egg
¾ cup honey
2¾ cups flour
1 teaspoon soda (not vanilla)
1 teaspoon salt
1 teaspoon lemon flavouring

Cream shortening and sugar. Add egg and mix well. Add honey and beat until well mixed. Sift together the flour, soda and salt. Add to the mixture on low speed then add lemon flavouring. Mix only until blended. Chill the dough. Roll out and cut into shapes. Grease baking sheet. Bake at 190°C (375°F, gas mark 5) for 8-10 minutes until a very light golden colour. Frost as desired.

Mushrooms in Red Wine

Ingredients:

175g wild mushrooms
175g button mushroom
175g oyster mushroom
3 garlic cloves
4 tablespoons red wine
1 tablespoon fresh parsley, chopped
1 tablespoon fresh chives, chopped
2 tablespoons olive oil
salt and ground black pepper for seasoning

Peel and thinly slice the cloves of garlic. Clean the mushrooms, remove the stalks and slice or quarter the mushrooms. Heat the olive oil in a large frying pan. When hot, sauté the garlic then add the mushrooms and cook until they have softened. Stir in the red wine and fresh herbs. Season according to taste with salt and black pepper. Continue cooking until the juices have thickened. Serve with hot French bread.